# MEDICAL CODING

## STUDY GUIDE AND TRAINING TOOL

# MEDICAL CODING

## STUDY GUIDE AND TRAINING TOOL

IN POPULAR QUESTION AND ANSWER FORMAT
COMPLIES WITH THE LATEST CODING STANDARD

- A Rigorous Study Guide to Prepare for Certification Exams
- A Training Tool - Better Accuracy and Speed
- A Must Have Guide for All AAPC, AHIMA and MMI Coding Certification Examinations

**CODING METHODOLOGIES AND PRACTICAL CASES FOR**

Surgery | Cardiology | Pulmonology | Orthopedic Surgery | Plastic Surgery
Pain management | OB-GYN | Anesthesiology

**Vino C. Mody Jr., MD, PhD**
Consultant and Trainer in Healthcare and Medical Administration Processes
Certified in Medical Coding for All fields

Suwanee Press
www.SuwaneePress.com

Suwanee Press
www.SuwaneePress.com

 The book is complaint with the 2019 codebooks ICD-10-CM, CPT, HCPCS II and 2018 ASA Crosswalk(R) and 2019 Relative Value Guide(R).

First Printing: 2019

ISBN-13: 978-1-947333-04-8

Suwanee Press
1115 River Laurel Dr.
Suwanee, Georgia, 30024

www.SuwaneePress.com
This book can be ordered from Amazon

Synopsis of

# *A Medical Coding Study Guide and Training Tool*

By

Vino Mody Jr., MD, PhD

Medical coding for insurance purposes would seem, on the surface, to be a straightforward process that involves simple memorization of the codes for various medical procedures—or at least the ability to search out the codes in a database. However, as this book shows, medical procedures always involve individual patients who have their own medical idiosyncrasies that will, in almost all cases, defeat this simplistic approach to coding. Fast and prompt coding of medical procedures requires skill and knowledge, and the purpose of this book is to give medical coders the training they need today, in 2019, to be successful at what they do. The book is valuable both for readers who are facing the CANPC™ examinations and those who are already working as coders and wish to refresh their skills.

This book goes beyond a mere listing of codes and instead focuses on providing insights into the multitude of scenarios that coders face when presented with actual medical cases. The book utilizes a popular question-and-answer format to explore 50 unique medical cases that simulate an actual CANPC™ examination. The book highlights the correct coding method and provides the reader with invaluable practice in applying coding principles to actual real-life patient cases. Each case is then provided with a solution that lists the best coding decision for that patient scenario. Every case is also discussed from a clinical viewpoint to explain the rationale underlying the different coding decisions and the generation of Medicare coding units for that patient.

This book will be an invaluable asset for anyone working in, or planning to work in, the medical coding field.

The acronyms AAPC, AHIMA and MMI are used in the title and throughout the book. These are well-known to healthcare organizations and employees, however, for clarity, these acronyms are deciphered here:

| | | |
|---|---|---|
| AAPC | – | American Academy of Professional Coders |
| AHIMA | – | American Health Information Management Association |
| MMI | – | Medical Management Institute |

# Contents

# Dedication

Dedicated to my parents, my brother, and my uncle Manoj Shah; MD,
a practicing OBG and former president of AMA, Georgia Chapter,
for their support and encouragement

# Acknowledgments

I would like to express my gratitude to several individuals within healthcare institutions and the local chapter of the American Academy of Professional Coders (AAPC) in El Paso, Texas for their guidance and opportunities provided for learning, teaching, and networking with healthcare professionals in Texas. My sincere thanks to:

Yasenia Ceniceros, an instructor, and supervisor at Southwest University

Ms. Ellen Eastman, President of AAPC Local Chapter

Roberta Pell, organizer of Local Chapter events and proctor for examinations for various healthcare related certifications.

I learned a lot from the teaching sessions I conducted and presentations by administrative professionals at the local AAPC chapter and educational institutes. I appreciate the guidance I received from Kathleen Cahill, CEO of Mesa Hills Specialty Hospital in El Paso, where I worked for over a year in medical administrative functions.

I wish to offer special thanks to my father, Vino Mody, for his excellent help with the editing of this book and for coordinating with the designer and publisher to get the book ready for production.

I am very grateful to Mr. Mark Schutte, Senior Communications Network Consultant, in Suwanee, GA for his guidance on the publication process and direct help in the book layout and release of its hard copy and eBook.

The author gratefully acknowledges that the sources listed in the Reference section of this book were modified and used stating the cases, and sincerely thanks the publishers of these sources. The author recommends that students preparing for medical coding certification examinations study these references.

# Preface

This book presents and elaborates fundamental principles about medical coding for several areas of specialty and how to approach coding accurately and efficiently. The book covers key steps for coding and a correct method for determining the overall code for each case. This study guide with problems and solutions covers all areas of medical coding, including general surgery, cardiology, pulmonology, orthopedic surgery, plastic surgery, pain management, OB-GYN and anesthesiology. The book borrows some of the details for the cases (problems) from other sources disclosed in References; these are further elaborated by the author with his knowledge as a physician to present a cross section of a balanced variety of situations helpful to a coding student and practitioner. Included in the book are many useful topics: unit calculations, anesthesia and pain management modifiers, physical status, and qualifying circumstances—or what the author calls emergency conditions, and clinical viewpoints for each case. The presentation is concisely written to get the point across in an effective way making the subject of the book easier to understand and explain. The book comprises of 50 comprehensive cases discussed to teach details of coding techniques.

The book is a clear guide for people who would like to learn medical coding or refresh their skills. The book is structured as a tutorial and is a useful 2019 supplement to the 2018 coding study guide the author published in 2018 (ISBN: 978-1-947333-02-4); it will be valuable in your employee training programs for general coding.

The best and proven successful approach to becoming well-versed in medical coding is to learn the basic concept of coding and medical terminology and, last but not least, to practice. He author recommends that you read the introductory paragraphs and then complete cases 1 through 50, and then compare your answers with the solutions for each case offered at the end of the book.

The medical coding exams are challenging and require substantial preparation. General coding involves complex terminology that you must learn, apart from the coding techniques. In fact, your coding speed and precision would depend on your understanding of medical terminology, which you can learn from several affordable sources. The book is good preparation for several medical coding certification exams offered by AAPC and AHIMA. In addition, AAPC, AHIMA, Medical Management Institute, and The American Society of Medical Coding provide learning material contained in their magazines and lectures; you may wish to refer to these sources. This book will be extremely helpful in preparing and passing several medical coding certification exams important for the career of medical coders, as follows.

<u>Certification exams from AAPC</u>

Professional Coder (CPC™)

Inpatient Coder (CIC™)

Ambulatory Surgical Center (CASCC™)

Cardiology Coder (CCC™)

Outpatient Coder (COC™)

Risk Adjustment Coder (CRC™)

Anesthesia and pain management (CANPC™)

Cardiovascular/Thoracic Surg.Coder (CCVTC™)

Emergency Department Coder(CEDC™)
Evaluation Management Coder (CEMC™) Interven.
Radiology/Cardiovascular (CIRCC™)
Obstetrics and Gynecology Coder (COBGC™)
Urology Coder (CUC™)
Orthopedic surgery Coder (COSC™)

Certification exams from AHIMA

Coding Associate (CCA)
Coding Specialist (CCS)
Coding Specialist-Physician Based (CCS-P)

Certification exams from MMI

Registered medical coder (RMC)
Regd. Evaluation/MGMT Specialist (REMS).

The local chapter of the AAPC nearest to your town may have periodic conferences attended by coders, coding teachers and experienced professional; it is highly recommended the aspiring medical coders should attend.

# The Book Outline

*A Medical Coding Study Guide and Training Tool*

By

Vino Mody Jr., MD, PhD

The aim of this book is to provide the reader with the latest 2019 standard in medical coding for several areas of specialty in a popular question-and-answer style. The aim of the book is threefold: it serves as a rigorous study guide for healthcare workers who are preparing for coding certification examinations, it acts as a training tool to allow coders to improve their speed and accuracy in real-life coding situations, and it provides an overview of the AAPC, AHIMA, and MMI coding certification exams. Its goal is to present coding methodologies and practical cases for medical areas ranging from surgery and cardiology to anesthesiology and OB-GYN. The author, Vino C. Mody, MD, PhD, shares his many years of expertise in medical coding to provide a hands-on study guide that gives the reader real-life coding scenarios that raise the coding aptitude of the reader well beyond just the ability to memorize codes.

The book breaks down the coding issues according to each anatomical system, covering the integumentary, musculoskeletal, respiratory, cardiovascular, urinary, male and female reproductive, endocrine, and nervous systems. The book also provides 50 actual coding problems, based on actual hospital case scenarios, for the readers to test their own abilities to provide the correct code for complex cases, thereby training the readers to provide codes easily and accurately when faced with any real-life patient scenario. The book gives the readers the option of working through each of the 50 cases one-by-one, and checking the solutions provided at the end of the book, to understand the clinical viewpoints that explain the rationale underlying different coding decisions. The readers gain much needed practice in coding, which will benefit both those preparing for the difficult medical coding exams and those who simply wish to refresh their skills in the real-life complexities of medical coding situations.

# Introduction

This book shows how to generate accurate codes for each individual medical case discussed. It also helps the coders, billers, and other workers in healthcare organizations to prepare for various coding examinations as listed in an earlier section Preface. The book gives the reader essentially "real-life" practice in coding, with all the "real-life" complexities that you know the coder will encounter someday. Learning the concepts and applications by practicing on a large number of exercises—as included in books like this written by subject matter experts—is necessary if you are to attain the desired speed and accuracy in the coding process. Equally importantly, the healthcare management can also use the book for training and retraining of medical coders employees. Of course, the ultimate level of competency will come from the wealth of knowledge offered in books like this combined with working under experienced mentors, as in any field.

The book will immensely help professionals taking the coding certification examinations conducted by AAPC, AHIMA and MMI (Medical Management Institute). The 50 cases highlight principles outlined in this study guide, and elaborate on 2019 coding procedure according to the American Academy of Professional Coders. Notably, the clinical viewpoints (*from a physician's perspective*) are offered throughout the book as appropriate, and these cover the rationale for the coding decisions made in cases discussed.

Medical diagnosis and treatment procedures are complex, and they demand understanding, experience and expertise working with medical diagnosis and treatment details. Correct, proper and prompt coding is crucial in insurance approval of payments for the services provided to patients. Wrong or unclear codes delay insurance payments. Worse yet, the wrong codes can raise potential legal problems for the healthcare company if the payer notes a history of excessive billed amounts over and above the allowed amounts for given services.

Coding certifications from AAPC, AHIMA and MMI adds significantly to your credentials and credibility when working with billers and insurance companies, and it ultimately helps your employer, whether a private medical practice or a hospital. The membership with AAPC and AHIMA expands your contact network with other coding practitioners and supports your credibility as a professional coder.

Relevant topics of diagnostic coding for various medical fields such as *general surgery, cardiology, pulmonology, orthopedic surgery, plastic surgery, pain management, OB-GYN and anesthesiology* are reviewed in the book. As a prerequisite to passing a coding examination, you must know how to derive the appropriate ICD-10-CM codes per the 2019 standard and the right sequencing of diagnostic codes, particularly when multiple codes are required to assess the actual disease condition. Note all coding examinations permit you to have the ASA Crosswalk®, Relative Value Guide®, and an audit worksheet with you for reference.

The discussion on every case highlights the correct method of coding, and thus enhancing your chance for success on the said certification exams. The material herein also helps you as a coder in your ability to do accurate work by giving you additional practice and apply the coding principles to actual cases. Knowing the details regarding how to perform coding is imperative obviously for passing the exam. The author believes strongly that by following the instructions taught in this book will enable you to come up with correct codes.

# Anesthesia and pain management coding

## CPT Coding methodologies

CPT coding discipline requires that you follow a structured process. Anesthesiology coding is not straightforward and requires attention to details. I have developed a universally applied formal method for determining the overall anesthesia code for a case. The following are my recommended steps for anesthesia coding that I encourage you to follow:

### Step 1: Determine the appropriate anesthesia code for the surgical procedures provided, utilizing the ASA Crosswalk Lookup

For example, the corresponding anesthesia code for CPT code 66984 Extracapsular cataract removal with insertion of intraocular lens prosthesis (1 stage procedure), manual or mechanical technique is 00142 Anesthesia for procedures on eye; lens surgery. CPT code=base value units= (corresponding) anesthesia code; 66984=4 base value units=00142

The method for anesthesiology coding is outlined later in this book, under that title.

For two or more CPT codes, select the overall anesthesia code with highest base value units. For a tie, select the anesthesia code that corresponds to the first-listed CPT code.

### Step 2: Assign modifiers to identify the anesthesia provider

The modifiers for the provider can be either for the anesthesiologist (or doctor) or for the CRNA(s). Distinguishing between Anesthesiologist or Doctor and CRNA modifier codes is important. Anesthesiologist or Doctor codes are for the billing anesthesiologist, whereas CRNA codes are for the billing CRNA.

See the table in HCPCS II.

- AA [Anesthesiologist] Anesthesia services performed personally by anesthesiologist
- AD [Anesthesiologist] Medical supervision by a physician; more than four concurrent anesthesia procedures [more than 4 CRNAs is included here]
- QK [Doctor] Medical direction of two, three, or four concurrent anesthesia procedures involving qualified individuals [2, 3, or 4 CRNAs is included here]
- QS Monitored anesthesia care (MAC) service
- QX [CRNA] CRNA service: with medical direction by a physician
- QY [Doctor] Medical direction of one certified registered nurse anesthetist (CRNA) by an anesthesiologist
- QZ [CRNA] CRNA service: without medical direction by a physician

### Step 3: Report physical status modifiers for anesthesia services

PS I through PS VI can be found in the Relative Value Guide®. The base units for each physical status are important in the unit calculation for PS or physical status. PS with corresponding base unit values is listed.

- P1: A normal healthy patient= 0
- P2: A patient with mild systemic disease= 0
- P3: A patient with severe systemic disease= 1
- P4: A patient with severe systemic disease that is a constant threat to life= 2
- P5: A moribund patient who is not expected to survive without the operation= 3
- P6: A declared brain-dead patient whose organs are being removed for donor purposes= 0

## Step 4: Report qualifying circumstance codes when appropriate

I call qualifying circumstances codes by the heading Emergency.

Qualifying circumstances with base unit values

- +99100: Anesthesia for a patient of extreme age, younger than 1 year and older than 70= 1
- +99116: Anesthesia complicated by utilization of total body hypothermia= 5
- +99135: Anesthesia complicated by utilization of controlled hypotension= 5
- +99140: Anesthesia complicated by emergency conditions= 2

## Field avoidance and special positioning with base unit values

"Field avoidance" means the anesthesia provider does not have access to the patient's airway during surgery. Any procedure around the head, neck, or shoulder girdle that requires field avoidance, or any procedure requiring a position other than supine or lithotomy, has a minimum base unit value of 5, regardless of any lesser base value assigned to such a procedure in the body of the Relative Value Guide®.

Code additional procedures performed by the anesthesia provider. To count as a separately reportable code on the anesthesiology service, note that the anesthesia provider has to perform the additional procedures, not the surgeon.

To be clear, the following procedures are separately reported for the anesthesiology service if performed by the anesthesiology provider (Anesthesiologist or Doctor or CRNA)

- Insertion of central venous catheters: 36555 or 36556
- Insertion of arterial catheters: 36620 or 36625
- Insertion of Swan Ganz catheter: 93503
- Transesophageal echocardiogram (TEE): 93312

## Determine the total units for anesthesia services

For unit calculations, you can use:

- Units = Base + Time + PS + Emergency

Base units (for the anesthesia code), time units (anesthesia time/15), PS (physical status modifier) units, and Emergency (Qualifying circumstances) units are added together to generate the total units.

- Medicare units = Base + Time (For a Medicare patient)

## Method for anesthesiology coding

The method for determining the overall anesthesiology code for a case is structured and universally applicable. The method involves utilization of the ASA Crosswalk® and looking at the base value units for each procedure.

## Anesthesiology coding

To determine the overall anesthesia code for a case, look up each CPT code in the ASA (American Society of Anesthesiologists) Crosswalk and note the corresponding anesthesiology code with its base unit value. Note that the anesthesiology code with the highest base unit value is the overall anesthesia code for the case for all CPT procedures.

Example:

Anesthesia services provided by an anesthesiologist (PS III)

Arstasis: Introduce access device for self-sealing arteriotomy; Enlarged aneurysm area near the anastomosis to the brachial artery, excise the AV fistula

CPT and ICD-10-CM codes:

- 35011, 35206, 37607, I71.2

## Corresponding anesthesia codes with base unit values and CPT codes

ASA Crosswalk Lookup

- 35011 = 10 base value units = 01652
- 35206 = 4 base value units = 01782
- 37607 = 6 base value units = 01840

In order to select the overall anesthesia code for this case, choose the anesthesia code with the highest base value units; note that the first listed code splits a tie.

- 01652-AA-P3

## Types of anesthesia

Several types of anesthesia are available, depending on how deep the anesthesia for the case should be and whether the anesthesia involves the entire body, a region, or only a small area.

### Local

- Local anesthesia is bundled with the minor surgery CPT code

### Monitored anesthesia care (MAC)

- Deep sedation, in which the patient can respond to painful stimuli but maintains control of the airway

### Regional

- Epidurals and nerve blocks
- Provides anesthesia for a region of the body

## General

- The patient is unconscious and has no control of the airway

## Services included in the anesthesia code for general anesthesia, MAC, or regional anesthesia

The following services are included:

- Pre-operative visits, post-operative visits, patient care during the procedure, administration of fluids and blood, EKGs, temperature measurement, blood pressures, intubation, laryngoscopy, introduction of a needle or catheter, venipuncture, blood transfusions, blood sample procurement through an existing line, temporary transcutaneous pacemakers, and injections of diagnostic or therapeutic substances.

### Obstetric anesthesia

Obstetric anesthesia is anesthesia provided during labor and delivery for a woman. When selecting a code for obstetric anesthesia, check to see if the patient had received neuraxial labor analgesia prior to delivery for pain control and anesthesia. Report 01967 for neuraxial labor analgesia/anesthesia for planned vaginal delivery, including any repeat subarachnoid needle placement and drug injection as well as any necessary replacement of an epidural catheter during labor.

### Daily Hospital Management of an Epidural

Daily hospital management of an epidural is reported starting with the first postoperative day (01996) and not on the day of the epidural or subarachnoid catheter placement.

### Trigger point injections

In a trigger point injection, a local anesthetic is injected into a trigger point to relieve pain in a muscle. It is counted based on the number of muscles injected, not the number of injections (20552)).

### Sacroiliac injection

Sacroiliac injection of anesthetic or steroid utilizing CT or fluoroscopy imaging guidance is included in 27096.

### Discography

Discography is performed to see if a disc is the source of a patient's pain. Contrast is injected into the disc, and the patient's response to the injection is documented. Discography (62290 or 62291) combined with radiological supervision and interpretation (72285 or 72295) is performed with contrast injected into the disc.

### Epidurals

- Single injection not via an indwelling catheter (coded 62310 or 62311)
- Injection, including catheter placement, for continuous infusion of intermittent bolus (coded 62318 or 62319)
- When the epidural is the method for the anesthesia, code the appropriate anesthesia (coded 00100–01999)

### Transforaminal epidural

CPT codes are based on the number of levels and region of the spine and are performed for diagnostic and therapeutic purposes.

- The procedure (64479 -64484) can identify which nerve is causing the pain, and it can be performed for chronic pain.
- If the provider performs ultrasound guidance, code Category III codes as 0228T or 0229T; 0230T, or 0231T.

### Pain pumps

Procedures for pain pumps are used for pain management or spasticity treatment are reported with codes 62350–62370.

When an intrathecal or epidural catheter is connected to an implantable reservoir or an implantable infusion pump (IIP), codes 62350 or 62351 are reported.

Programmable infusion pumps (PIIP) and IIPs are important for drug delivery systems and for treatment of a wide range of clinical conditions, such as cancer and chronic pain.

### Facet joint injections

Facet joint injections temporarily relieve pain by filling the facet joint with an anesthetic medication that numbs the facet joint and the ligaments and joint capsule that surround the facet joint.

Facet joint injections are used for injections of diagnostic or therapeutic agents in paravertebral facet (zygapophyseal) joints (or nerves innervating that joint) with image guidance (fluoroscopy or CT); these are coded by 64490, 64491, 64492, 64493, 64494, or 64495, depending on the level of the injection. (For example, 64490 is used for cervical or thoracic; single level.)

### Nerve blocks

A nerve block is an injection of an anesthetic agent directly (64400–64455) near a nerve to stop the pain. When a nerve block is performed for regional anesthesia, report the appropriate anesthesia code (00100–01999).

### Destruction by a neurolytic agent

- Neurolytic agents destroy nerve tissue (64600–64640) for ongoing relief of pain for weeks or up to a year due to disease or other abnormality of the nerve root. This procedure is known as a rhizotomy.

### Relative value order

CPT codes should be arranged in relative value order, a concept applied in Certified Cardiovascular and Thoracic Surgery Coder (CCVTC) theory. Each CPT code has a relative valuc unit, as found in the 2017 National Physician Fee Schedule Relative Value File January Rclease, copyrighted in 2015 by the American Medical Association and in 2016/17 by the American Dental Association. The first-listed CPT code is the CPT code with the highest corresponding relative value unit, followed by the second-listed CPT code, which has the second highest relative value unit, and correspondingly in the same fashion to the last-listed CPT code, which has the lowest relative value unit. All CPT codes in this book are arranged in the correct relative value order, which is important for solving a split-tie in cases of anesthesia coding. In a case of a split-tie in anesthesia coding, the first-listed CPT code in the split-tie is the overall anesthesia code for the case.

### Cases for CANPC™ exam simulation

Discussed in the following are case numbers 1 through 50, which the readers need to practice and learn in order to prepare for the CANPC™ examination and to be better coders. Cases 1 through 50 are a CANPC™ simulation exam, which can help prepare candidates for the actual CANPC™ exam. The candidate should prepare for the CANPC™ exam by first studying AAPC's CANPC™ study guide and then taking the CANPC™ simulation exam (cases 1–50) outlined in this book. I recommend completing 7-8 cases per day, which is the length of the AAPC CANPC study guide. The CANPC™ simulation exam in this book is based on the actual exam, and it covers novel material not found elsewhere.

### Anatomical systems

#### *1. Integumentary System*

The skin is made up of two primary layers: the epidermis and dermis. The table of neoplasms is broken down into six columns: Primary, secondary, Ca is situ. Diseases of skin and subcutaneous tissue include skin infections, inflammatory conditions of the skin, and other disorders of the skin. Skin infections can be bacterial or fungal. Impetigo (L01) is caused by group A streptococci or Staphylococcus aureus entering the skin. Cutaneous abscesses, carbuncles, and furuncle (L02) can be caused by Staphylococcal infection. L02 is cellulitis and acute lymphangitis. A pilonidal cyst (L05) is a cyst, fistula, or sinus under the skin located at the bottom of the tailbone.

#### *1a. Integumentary System: CPT coding methodologies*

Now let us review a few CPT codes in this section. CPT coding in integumentary system includes incision and drainage (I&D) of an abscess, cyst, or hematoma (10060, 10061, 10080, 10081, 10140, and 10160). Debridement (11000-11008) is the removal of dead tissue.

### 2. Musculoskeletal System

Rheumatoid arthritis (M05) and osteoarthritis (M15-M19) are conditions of the musculoskeletal system. Joint derangement codes include tears or damage to cartilage or ligaments (M23.2). Systemic lupus erythematosus (M32), dorsopathies (M40-M54), rheumatism (M79.0), enthesopathies (M77.9), synovitis (M65.9), tenosynovitis (M65.9), bursitis (M71.9), osteopathies and chondropathies, osteomyelitis (M86.9), osteoporosis and pathological fractures (M80.00), and hallux valgus or other deformities of toes (M20.1-) are conditions of the musculoskeletal system. A closed fracture has not broken the skin and an open fracture is where the bone is protruding through the skin. Injuries are the cause of Compartment Syndrome. Compartment syndrome (T79.7, T79.A0) is the compression of nerves and blood vessels within an enclosed space. The four muscles of the rotator cuff (supraspinatus, infraspinatus, subscapularis, and teres minor muscles) are attached to the scapula through a single tendon unit. Rotator cuff tears (M75.10-) occur in sports. Toddlers present with Nursemaid's elbow (S53.03-). A fracture can be comminuted, impacted, simple, Greenstick, pathologic, compression, or torus or incomplete. External cause codes or located in the External Cause of Injuries Index and capture how the injury or health condition happened (cause), the intent (unintentional, accidental, or intentional), the place where the event occurred, the activity of the patient, and the patient's status (civilian or military).

#### 2a. Musculoskeletal System: CPT coding methodologies

CPT coding in this section includes wound exploration for penetrating gunshot or stab wound trauma (20100-20103). Spinal surgery (22010-22899) is also included. Diagnostic arthroscopy is always included in therapeutic or surgical arthroscopy.

### 3. Respiratory, Hemic & Lymphatic Systems; Mediastinum, and Diaphragm

Acute respiratory infections include pneumonia and influenza (J09-J18), other diseases of the upper respiratory tract (J30-J39), chronic lower respiratory diseases (J40-J47), lung diseases due to external agents (J60-J70), respiratory failure (J96), other diseases of the respiratory system, symptoms, and Z codes. Mediastinum and diaphragm includes codes related to herniation of the diaphragm (K44), diaphragmatic paralysis (J98.6), thymic hyperplasia (E32.0), and thymoma, both benign (C79.89) and malignant (C37). Hemic and lymphatic systems includes codes related to lymphoma (C81-C88), lymphadenitis (I88, L04), lymphedema, acquired I89.0, I97.2, I97.89, or congenital Q82.0), disorders involving the immune mechanism (D80-D89), hypersplenism (D73.1), splenic rupture including rupture during birth (P15.1) and traumatic rupture (S36.09), leukemia (C91-C95), multiple myeloma (C90), leukemia in remission (Z85.6), and malignant neoplasms of lymphoid, hematopoietic, and related tissues (Z85.79).

#### 3a. Respiratory, Hemic & Lymphatic Systems; Mediastinum, and Diaphragm: CPT coding methodologies

CPT codes in the respiratory system consists of codes such as rhinoplasty including septoplasty (30400-30630), surgical endoscopies of accessory sinuses (31231-31298), laryngotomy (31300) or laryngectomy (31360-31382), bronchoscopy (31622-31654), and lymph node excision (38700-38780).

### 4. Cardiovascular System

Arrhythmias and conduction disorders include atrial fibrillation (I48.91), atrial flutter (I48.92), paroxysmal supraventricular tachycardia (PSVT) (I47.1), ventricular tachycardia (V-tach) (I47.2), ventricular fibrillation (V-fib) (I49.01), and bradycardia (R00.1). Hypertension (I10-I15) includes hypertension with heart disease (I11), which requires a causal link, hypertensive chronic kidney disease (I12), which has an assumed causal link, hypertensive heart and chronic kidney disease (I13), hypertensive cerebrovascular disease (I60-I69), hypertensive retinopathy (H35.0, I10-I15), secondary hypertension (I15), transient hypertension and elevated blood pressure (R03.0,), transient hypertension complicating pregnancy (O14), hypertension, controlled or uncontrolled (I10-I15), or hypertensive crisis (I16). Arteriosclerosis includes chronic ischemic heart disease (I25). Endocarditis (I33-I39) includes rheumatic endocarditis (I01, I09). More cardiovascular conditions include pericarditis (I30-I32), heart failure (I50), peripheral arterial disease (PAD) (I73), valve disorders (I05-I09, I34-I37), cerebrovascular accident (I60-I67, I69), myocardial infarction (MI) (I21-I22), intraoperative and postprocedural complications (I97), and anticoagulant therapy (Z79.01).

### *4a. Cardiovascular System: CPT coding methodologies*

Coronary artery bypass graft (33510-33536) is performed to bypass blockages in the coronary arteries to improve blood flow. Central venous access procedures (36555-36598) involve catheters placed in large veins for patients who require frequent access to the bloodstream.

A method for Coronary artery bypass grafting (CABG) for severe coronary artery disease is presented based on a case from 2016-2017 AHA Coding Clinic ICD-10-CM/PCS and HCPCS subscription. The method is applicable to proper cardiovascular coding for the CCVTC™ exam from AAPC. The relative value units were based on 2017 National Physician Fee Schedule Relative Value File January Release.

## Case

A 55 year old patient with type 2 diabetes mellitus and a smoker was admitted for coronary artery bypass graft (CABG) for treatment of severe coronary artery disease. He had symptoms of unstable angina including worsening chest pain and dyspnea. He also has significant peripheral vascular disease. Before CABG operation, patient underwent left and right heart catheterization including left ventriculography and coronary angiogram which showed 95% occlusion in the left anterior descending artery, 100% stenosis of the posterior descending artery, 90% occlusion in the diagonal artery, and 97% occlusion of the obtuse marginal artery. Ventriculography showed the heart to be of normal contractility with no dilation or dyskinetic action and with an ejection fraction of 65%.

**Place of service:** Hospital B

**Surgeon:** Dr. D

**Assistant surgeon:** Dr. B

**Preoperative diagnosis:** Coronary artery disease

**Postoperative diagnosis:** Severe coronary artery disease with > 90% occlusion in LAD, posterior descending artery, diagonal artery, and obtuse marginal artery

**Operation:** Aortocoronary bypass grafting times four with implantation of left inferior mammary artery (LIMA) and left anterior descending (LAD) coronary artery; Separate saphenous vein bypass graft from the aorta to the posterior descending artery, obtuse marginal artery, and diagonal artery; endoscopic vein harvest.

### *Method*

Determine whether the coronary bypass is venous grafting only, combined arterial-venous grafting, or arterial grafting only. Determine the number of venous and arterial grafts in a matrix. Determine the overall CPT codes for the case.

### *Matrix*

### *Grafting*

-→ Posterior descending artery (a branch of right coronary artery)

Saphenous vein -→ Obtuse marginal (a branch of left circumflex artery)

-→ Diagonal (a branch of left coronary artery)

LIMA -→ LAD

Vino C. Mody Jr., COC, CPC, CCS-P, CANPC, CCVTC

### Codes

33533, 93460, +33519, +33508, I25.110, E11.51, F17.200

Relative value units, used in CPT coding to determine rank order of CPT codes (highest RVU is listed first)

93460, RVU=34.13

33533, RVU-54.22

33519, RVU=15.83

33508, RVU=0.47

In this case, there is combined arterial and venous grafting. There are 3 venous grafts and one arterial graft. The patient underwent endoscopic vein harvest of the saphenous vein. The patient has atherosclerotic heart disease of native coronary artery with unstable angina pectoris. The patient has type 2 diabetes mellitus and is a smoker, which increase the chance of developing coronary artery disease. He also has peripheral vascular disease which is reflective of atherosclerotic vessel disease peripherally in this case of severe coronary artery disease requiring four-vessel CABG.

## 5. Urinary System and Male Genital System

Diseases of the genitourinary system (N00-N99) include nephritis, pyelonephritis (N10-N12), hydronephrosis (N13), and renal failure (N17-N19). Other diseases of the urinary system (N30-N39) include cystitis (N30), voiding disorders (N32), and urinary tract infection (N39). Diseases of the male genital organs (N40-N53) include benign hyperplasia of the prostate (BPH) (N40-), prostatitis (N41), dysplasia of the prostate (N42.30), and prostatic intraeplithelial neoplasia III (PIN III) (D07.5). Disorders of the spermatic cord, testis, tunica vaginalis, and epididymis include hydrocele (N43) and orchitis (N45.2). Penile disorders include phimosis (N47.1), balanitis (N48.1), balanoposthitis (N48), other inflammatory disorders of the penis and priapism (N48), vascular disorders (N48), edema, impotence (N48), and Peyronie's disease (N48). Congenital malformations of male genital organs include hypospadias (Q54) and epispadias (Q64.0). Genitourinary cancer diagnoses are found within the Neoplasm chapter of ICD-10-CM and are specific to the anatomy of the organ. Common genitourinary cancers are renal cell carcinoma (C64-C65), bladder cancer (C67), prostate cancer (C61), and testicular cancer (C62). Injuries to the genitourinary organs include injuries of the kidney, pelvic organs, and external genitalia (S30-S39). Symptoms and signs involving the genitourinary system are found in R30-R39.

### 5a. Urinary System and Male Genital System: CPT coding methodologies

CPT codes for the urinary system include of renal stones from the renal pelvis (50130-50135). CPT codes for the male genital system include vasectomy (55250) for birth control.

## 6. Female Reproductive System

Neoplasms of the female reproductive system can originate from the ovaries (C56), uterus (C55), cervix (C53.9), and vulva (C51.9). Leiomyoma (D25.9) are benign tumors. Conditions of the female genitourinary system include premenopausal menorrhagia (N92.4) and postmenopausal bleeding (N95.0). Diseases of the pregnancy include gestational diabetes (O24.4), normal delivery (O80), and supervision of a normal pregnancy (Z34).

### *6a. Female Reproductive System: CPT coding methodologies*

CPT coding of the female reproductive system includes excision of the vulva (56620-56640), which is performed for cancer. Laparoscopic lysis of adhesions of the oviducts and ovaries (58660) and tubal ligation (58600-58615) of the fallopian tubes.

### ***7. Endocrine and Nervous System***

Neoplasms in the endocrine system (C75.9) can include additional codes to indicate either functional activity by neoplasms and ectopic endocrine tissue or hyperfunction and hypofunction of endocrine glands associated with neoplasms. Disorders of the nervous system include meningitis (G03.9), encephalitis (G04.90), myelitis (G04.91), and encephalomyelitis (G04.90), organic sleep disorders (G47.9), pain (R52), migraine (G43.909), disorders of the peripheral nervous system (G64).

### *7a. Endocrine and Nervous System: CPT coding methodologies*

CPT coding in the endocrine system includes excision of the thyroid gland (60200-60271), adrenalectomy (60540-60545), and placement of intracranial neurostimulators (61850-61888). Injection (62320-62327), drainage (62272), or aspiration (62268) are CPT codes from the spine or spinal cord category.

# Problems

# CASE 1

## *Intraperitoneal*

**Date of Procedure:** XX/XX/XXXX

**Post-operative Diagnosis:** Sacral decubitus ulcer with a full-thickness skin loss ulcer involving necrosis of the subcutaneous tissue

**Procedure performed:** Sigmoid colostomy

**Surgeon:** Dr. Optum **Anesthesia:** General endotracheal **Estimated Blood Loss:** Minimal

Anesthesiologist, DM (the abbreviations of the doctor's name) personally provided the general endotracheal anesthesia for the case while directing two CRNAs, DX and PO (the abbreviations of the CRNAs' two names) (PS III)

CRNA placed a non-tunneled central venous catheter into the internal jugular vein at the beginning of the case

**Anesthesia time:** 3.17 hours beginning at instilling general endotracheal anesthesia and ending at recovery in the post-anesthesia care unit

**Indications for Procedure:** The patient is a 43-year-old female with a complicated recent medical history secondary to an anoxic brain injury from a fall from a horse. Patient already has undergone placement of a percutaneous endoscopic gastrostomy tube and tracheostomy but is currently presenting with a large sacral decubitus ulcer. The medical team caring for the ulcer feels that there is a need for colostomy for fecal diversion ulcer. The medical team caring for the ulcer feels that there is a need for a colostomy for fecal diversion to help the healing of this wound. This has been discussed in detail with the patient's family, including the possibility that the wound would not heal, given multiple medical problems. Risks, benefits, and alternatives were discussed with the patient's family, and informed consent was obtained.

**Operative Report:** After adequate general endotracheal anesthesia was obtained, the patient's abdomen was prepped and draped in the normal sterile fashion. A lower midline skin incision was made. Dissection was carried down through the extensive subcutaneous tissue to the fascia. The fascia and peritoneum were carefully opened. Upon entering the peritoneal cavity, the redundant portion of the sigmoid colon was visualized. The superior-most portion was identified, and it was divided with a GIA stapler. A small portion of the mesentery was divided to allow for mobilization. The sigmoid colon was mobilized along the left paracolic gutter. An area in the left lower quadrant was then identified for the colostomy. A skin incision was made, and again dissection was carried down through the extensive subcutaneous tissue to the fascia. The fascia and peritoneum were carefully opened, and sigmoid colon was brought out at this site in a good position. The fascia and peritoneum were closed using running double strand 0 PDS suture. The sigmoid colon was attached to the abdominal wall with interrupted 3-0 Vicryl and then the ostomy was matured, opening the distal end, entering it again with interrupted 3-0 Vicryl. Once it was completed, it was widely patent. An ostomy appliance and sterile dressings were applied. Sponge and needle counts were correct at the end of the procedure. The patient tolerated the procedure and was extubated and sent to the post-anesthesia care unit in stable condition.

# CASE 2

# Anorectal

**Post-operative diagnosis:** Excessive granulation tissue in the sinus tract as a remnant of previously excised pilonidal cyst

**Procedure Performed:** Anoscopy, exploration of sinus tract with instillation of methylene blue, wide excision of sinus tract and underlying granulation tissue

**Surgeon:** Dr. Optum

**Anesthesia:** General endotracheal

Anesthesiologist, GT personally provided the general endotracheal anesthesia for the case while concurrently directed three other procedures (PS III)

The anesthesia was complicated by utilization of controlled hypotension

**Anesthesia start time:** 8:02 A.M. **Anesthesia end time:** 9:07 A.M.

**Indications for Procedure:** Patient is a 42-year-old who says four months ago he noticed some yellow discharge in his underwear. He did not have much pain, just a little irritation in that area. He is status post excision of a pilonidal cyst. In the past and in the office on exam, it appeared this was going to be a fistula, as there was a punctate opening several centimeters from the anus at about the 10 to 11 o'clock position.

**Procedure:** With the patient prone jackknife, his perianal area was prepped and draped in sterile fashion. We then inspected the external anal area. At about 11 o'clock was a small opening in the skin, which was well healed. I could not express anything out of this and anoscopic exam did not reveal any significant pathology; no evidence of anal stenosis or fissures. I instilled methylene blue into the skin opening and none of the fluid entered the anal canal. I then was able to probe this for a distance medially and superiorly, and the overlying skin was opened over the probe and I found old scar and what appeared to be granulation tissue probably from his prior pilonidal cystectomy. I widely excised this area, cauterized any small bleeders, and we packed this open with one-inch iodoform gauze. I injected 0.5% Marcaine with epinephrine into the surrounding soft tissues, and a dressing was applied.

He tolerated the procedure well. Estimated blood loss was less than 10 ml. Sponge and needle counts were reported correct X2. There were no complications.

**Surgical Findings:** Probable old scar and granulation tissue, and maybe a small remnant of his old pilonidal cyst.

**Plan:** The patient will be discharged home on Percocet one to two p.o.q. 4h p.r.n. pain, 40 of these. He was instructed to get in the shower or tub twice a day and after each bowel movement. I will see him back in 1 to 2 weeks for follow-up.

CASE 3

# Upper gastrointestinal endoscopic

**Post-operative Diagnosis:** Removal of stents from biliary tree, s/p cholecystectomy

**Procedure Performed:** ERCP to remove stents

**Surgeon:** Dr. Optum

**Anesthesia:** General endotracheal

Anesthesiologist, MM personally provided the general endotracheal anesthesia for the case while directing one CRNA (PS III)

The surgeon placed an arterial catheter in the right radial artery prior to the beginning of the case

**Anesthesia start time:** 9:05 A.M. **Anesthesia end time:** 10:11 A.M.

**Indications for Procedure:** Stent removal following management of a cystic duct bile leak complicating laparoscopic cholecystectomy with the placement of overlapping fully covered biliary Wallflex stents.

**Description of Procedure:** After obtaining informed consent, the scope was passed under direct vision, Throughout the procedure, the patient's blood pressure, pulse, and oxygen saturation were monitored continuously. The ERCP was accomplished without difficulty. The patient tolerated the procedure well.

**Findings:** One stent originating in the biliary tree was emerging from the major papillae. The stent was patent. Two stents were removed from the biliary tree using a rat-toothed forceps. The bile duct was deeply cannulated with the 12 mm balloon. The contrast was injected. I personally interpreted the bile duct images. A cholecystectomy had been performed previously. The main bile duct, cystic duct, hepatic duct bifurcation, and left and right hepatic ducts and all intrahepatic branches were normal. The biliary tree was swept with a 12 mm balloon starting at the bifurcation. Nothing was found. The previous cystic duct bile leak has resolved.

**Impression:**

1. Two overlapping patent 10 mm by 6 cm and 4 cm fully covered biliary wallflex stent were removed
2. Normal common bile duct, cystic duct remnant, and intra-hepatic biliary system. S/P cholecystectomy with complete closure of previous cystic duct bile "leak"

**Recommendation:** Discharge patient to home (ambulatory). No restrictions in diet after this evening. Full liquids for the first meal late this afternoon.

# CASE 4

# *Hernia repairs*

**Post-operative Diagnosis:** Bilateral inguinal hernias
Small sebaceous cyst, left groin

**Procedure Performed:** Kugel mesh repair of bilateral inguinal hernias and excision of small sebaceous cyst of the left groin

**Surgeon:** Dr. Optum

**Anesthesia:** Monitored anesthesia care (MAC)

Two CRNAs, DS and PW personally provided the monitored anesthesia care for the case without direction by an anesthesiologist (PS II)

The Kugel mesh repair for bilateral inguinal hernias surgery was complicated by emergency bleeding.

**Anesthesia start time:** 11:27 A.M. **Anesthesia end time:** 1:18 P.M.

**Indications for Procedure:** The patient is a 43-year-old gentleman who works for a local moving company. He does a lot of work with a moving cart, experiences pain maneuvering it, and now has bilateral inguinal hernias. He is being admitted for repair. He also has a sebaceous cyst in the left groin area that has been painful, so this will be removed during the procedure as well.

**Description of Procedure:** The patient was brought to the operating room, the abdomen and external genitalia were prepped and draped in sterile fashion. One each side, mirror-like incisions were performed between the anterior superior iliac spine and pubic tubercle and were taken down to the external oblique that was divided in line with its fibers. The internal oblique muscle fibers were split, the transversalis fascia incised, and with blunt dissection, I dissected out the spermatic cord on both sides and this was looped with a Penrose drain. I dissected away two small indirect hernia sacs but he did have a direct hernia on the left and a small direct on the right. These were both repaired by inserting a small oval Kugel mesh to reach the public tubercle medially, cover Hasselbach's triangle anteriorly, Cooper's ligament inferiorly, and the internal ring laterally. This mesh was affixed to the tranversalis fascia with one 2-0 Vicryl suture, and soft tissues were injected with a 0.5% Marcaine with epinephrine. The external oblique on both sides was reapproximated with 2-0 Vicryl. Scarpa's layer and the skin were also closed with Vicryl as well. Steri-Strips and dressing were applied.

I then excised a 1 cm sebaceous cyst in the left groin area that has been bothering the patient. This was not inflamed but was elliptically excised and closed with three interrupted subcuticular Vicryl sutures. He tolerated these procedures well.

Estimated blood loss of 500 ccs. Sponge and needle counts reported correct x2. No complications.

**Findings:** Bilateral direct inguinal hernias and small sebaceous cyst left groin

# CASE 5

# Nerves, muscles, tendons, fascia, and bursae

**Date of Procedure:** XX/XX/XXXX

**Postoperative Diagnosis:** Right breast cancer; estrogen receptor (+)

**Procedure:** Right lumpectomy with needle localization and sentinel node biopsy

**Surgeon:** Dr. Optum

**Anesthesia:** General endotracheal

Anesthesiologist, MS personally directed the general endotracheal anesthesia for the case while running five other procedures concurrently (PS IV)

Anesthesiologist placed a radial arterial catheter in the patient prior to the beginning of the case

**Anesthesia start time:** 04:29 A.M. **Anesthesia end time:** 8:05 A.M.

**Estimated Blood Loss:** Minimal

**Specimen:** Right lumpectomy and right axillary sentinel node

**Indications for Procedure:** The patient is a 58-year-old female who had a biopsy positive for estrogen receptor (+) right breast cancer. Risks, benefits, and alternatives of lumpectomy were discussed with the patient and her husband, and informed consent was obtained.

**Description of Procedure:** A sentinel node injection was performed by radiology as was a needle localization. The patient was brought to the operating room and placed under general endotracheal anesthesia. Her right breast and axilla were prepped and draped in the usual sterile fashion. A curvilinear skin incision was made in the upper outer breast above the site of the mass, as marked radiology. The guidewire was lateral to this. A superior flap was created using electrocautery. An inferior flap was then created, again going down to the chest wall. Then going from medial and lateral, the lumpectomy specimen from the upper outer quadrant was dissected free up off the chest wall. Once the specimen was completely freed up, it appeared that the mass or hematoma cavity was in the central portion of the specimen. A guidewire was used to mark the lateral aspect. A silk suture was placed medially, and a Vicryl suture was placed superiorly. The lumpectomy specimen was then sent to radiology where it was confirmed that the clip was in the specimen. The lumpectomy specimen was then closed re-approximating the breast tissue with interrupted 3-0 Vicryl. The skin was closed with a running 4-0 Prolene. It should be noted that there were appropriate in vivo and ex vivo counts using Neoprobe on the lumpectomy specimen.

Once the lumpectomy was closed, the hot spot was identified in the right axilla and small skin incision was made. Then using the Neoprobe I was able to dissect what appeared to be a single sentinel lymph node. This was completely dissected free. It was marked for the pathologist, and the frozen section was obtained. I again had appropriate in vivo and ex vivo counts using the Neoprobe. There were no other hot spots or significant activity noted in the axilla. The frozen section came back as negative.

Once this determined, the axillary tissue was re-approximated with interrupted 3-0 Vicryl, and the skin was closed with running 4-0 Prolene. Marcaine 0.5% was injected along both the lumpectomy and axillary biopsy site. Sterile dressings were applied. Sponge and needle counts were correct at the end of the procedure.

The patient tolerated the procedure well, was extubated and sent to the post-anesthesia care unit in stable condition.

# CASE 6

## Intraperitoneal

Pre-operative diagnosis: Adenocarcinoma of the colon

**Post-operative diagnosis:** Adenocarcinoma of the transverse colon, no noted metastases

Procedure performed: Laparoscopic transverse colectomy

**Surgeon:** Dr. Optum

**Anesthesia:** General endotracheal with epidural

Anesthesiologist, DD personally provided the general endotracheal anesthesia for the case while directing one CRNA (PS IV)

During the case, there was emergency blood loss as a complication

Anesthesiologist personally placed a central venous catheter without tunneling into the right internal jugular vein of the patient prior to the beginning of the case

**Anesthesia start time:** 2:00 P.M. **Anesthesia end time:** 5:27 P.M.

Estimated blood loss: 1000 cc

### Operative Report

The 69-year old patient was brought to the operating room and had an epidural catheter placed. She was induced and intubated. She was re-positioned in a low lithotomy position in Allen stirrups and had a Foley catheter and orogastric tube placed for decompression. Pneumatic compression hose was placed prior to the induction of anesthesia and remained on throughout the procedure to prevent thrombosis and possible embolism. The patient was prepped and draped in a sterile fashion. An infraumbilical vertical incision was made in the skin for the camera port. The umbilicus was retracted anteriorly using Backhaus towel forceps. The Verss needle was passed through the midline abdominal fascia into the peritoneal cavity, and the peritoneal cavity was insufflated with carbon dioxide, maintained at a pressure of 15 mm Hg. The Optiview camera port was passed into the peritoneal cavity. The patient has had previous abdominal surgeries, so there were adhesions of the omentum to the midline wound, which also tethered the transverse colon to the midline wound.

The abdomen was carefully inspected laparoscopically. There was India ink in the left colon, and this was initially thought to be the site of the tumor. Adhesions were taken down from the splenic flexure and also the hepatic flexure was exposed, but there was no sight of India ink in any of these locations. The transverse colon could be observed laparoscopically from the hepatic flexure to its point of midline adhesions and also from the splenic flexure to the point of midline adhesion but could not be completely visualized in the midline. We judged that the site of the tumor was likely located in the area of the adhesions at the midline wound.

The infraumbilical portion of the midline wound was opened sharply through the skin and was carried through subcutaneous tissue and midline abdominal fascia with electrocautery. Adhesions of the omentum were taken down under direct vision with electrocautery. The site showed the India ink tattoo and palpable colon cancer. Sites were selected proximally and distally to the tumor where the transverse colon was cleaned with electrocautery.

The transverse mesocolon was harvested, resecting adjacent mesentery and lymph-bearing tissue. The associated omentum was also excised. The transverse colon was reconstructed over Dennis clamps with interrupted 4-0 silk sutures utilizing RB-1 needles in the usual fashion. At the completion of the anastomosis, there was no tension, and both limbs of bowel showed no evidence of ischemia. The lumen of the anastomosis was widely patent by palpation. The anastomosis was returned to the abdomen.

Midline abdominal fascia was closed with running 0 PDS suture, and the skin was closed with subcuticular 4-0 Monocryl suture. The 5 mm port sites that were placed in the left mid-abdomen and in the suprapubic area were closed with subcuticular 4-0 Monocryl. Benzoin and Steri-Strips were used to dress all skin incisions. Instrument and sponge counts were correct. Estimated blood loss was 1000 ml. The patient awoke from general anesthesia and was taken to the recovery area in good condition.

CASE 7

# Moderation sedation

**Pre-operative Diagnosis:** Spontaneous right-sided pneumothorax

**Post-operative Diagnosis:** Spontaneous right-sided pneumothorax

**Procedure Performed:** Placement of right-sided 20 French chest tube

**Surgeon:** Dr. Optum

**Anesthesia:** 1% lidocaine with epinephrine. IV morphine and Versed.

Anesthesiologist, HS personally provided the moderate conscious sedation for the case who was a different doctor than the surgeon who performed the placement of right-sided 20 French chest tube (PS II).

**Anesthesia start time:** 8:00 A.M. **Anesthesia end time:** 8:32 A.M.

**Indications for Procedure:** The patient is a 20-year-old male with spontaneous right-sided pneumothorax. Risks, benefits, and alternatives of right-sided chest tube placement were discussed with the patient and his mother, and informed consent was obtained.

**Operative Report**

IV sedation was given, using appropriate monitoring and nasal cannula oxygen. The patient's right chest was then prepped with Betadine. The area of a previous chest tube was anesthetized with 10 ml of 1% lidocaine with epinephrine. Then using a #11 blade, a small skin incision was re-opened.

Dissection was carried down through scar and subcutaneous tissue onto the chest wall, and the appropriate area along the chest wall was anesthetized again with another 10 ml of 1% lidocaine with epinephrine. The right chest was then entered above the adjacent to rib space with a Kelly clamp. There was a gush of air. A 20 French chest tube was placed without difficulty. It was hooked to suction. The chest tube was secured to the skin with interrupted 0 silk sutures. A 4 X 4 dressing was applied.

The patient tolerated the procedure well. A portable chest x-ray was pending at the time of dictation.

## CASE 8

# Intraperitoneal

**Pre-operative Diagnosis:** Carcinoma of the stomach

**Post-operative Diagnosis:** Carcinoma of the stomach; small tumors in the left lobe of the liver

**Surgeon:** Dr. Optum

**Procedure Performed:** Exploratory laparotomy with wedge biopsy of the liver

**Anesthesia:** General endotracheal

Anesthesiologist performed the general endotracheal anesthesia for the case while directing two CRNAs (P4)

Anesthesiologist placed a Swan-Ganz catheter in the patient at the beginning of the case

**Anesthesia start time:** 9:15 P.M.

The anesthesia start time began when the anesthesiologist placed the Swan-Ganz catheter at the beginning of the case.

The anesthesia for the case was complicated by controlled hypotension.

**Anesthesia end time:** 12:05 A.M. the following day

**Indications for Procedure:** This 72-year-old male patient was admitted to the general surgery service for a thorough G.I. work-up carried out because of the history of 60 lb. weight loss during the past eight months. GI series demonstrated a large space-occupying lesion in the fundus of the stomach. Chest films, liver scan, and diagnostic studies did not indicate metastatic spread. Therefore, it was elected to explore this patient; today was taken to the operating room.

**Description of Procedure:** Under general endotracheal anesthesia, the abdomen was prepped and draped in sterile fashion for an upper midline incision. A small upper midline incision was made to explore the abdomen. The peritoneum was entered. Manuel exploration demonstrated a large, hard, fixed mass on the posterior wall of the fundus of the stomach. These were small tumors noted in the left lobe of the liver. A node was selected for biopsy, and a small wedge of this was removed. The midline was then closed with interrupted figure-eight sutures of 0-stainless steel wire; retention sutures were utilized to close the same. The skin was closed with 3-0 black silk, and no blood was administered during the surgical procedure. The patient tolerated the procedure well.

CASE 9

# Upper gastrointestinal endoscopic

**Pre-operative Diagnosis:** Esophageal dysphagia, history of Ivor-Lewis resection for adenocarcinoma

**Post-operative Diagnosis:** Esophageal dysphagia, history of Ivor-Lewis resection for adenocarcinoma

**Procedure Performed:** Upper GI endoscopy with dilatation

**Anesthesia:** General endotracheal

Anesthesiologist, BN performed the general endotracheal anesthesia for the case while directing one CRNA (PS IV)

The surgeon placed a central venous catheter, non-tunneled into the left internal jugular vein at the beginning of the case

**Anesthesia start time:** 7:00 A.M. **Anesthesia end time:** 8:02 A.M.

Medications Given: Midazolam 7 mg IV

**Complications:** No immediate complications

**Description of Procedure:** After obtaining informed consent from the 70-year old patient, the endoscope was passed under direct vision. Throughout the procedure, the patient's blood pressure, pulse, and oxygen saturation were monitored continuously. The endoscope was introduced through the mouth and advanced to the third part of the duodenum to complete the dilatation. The upper GI endoscopy was accomplished without difficulty. The patient tolerated the procedure well.

A benign-appearing, intrinsic mild esophagogastric anastomotic stricture measuring 2 cm (in length) x 1.2 cm (inner diameter) was found 37 cm from the incisors and traversed. The gastric body, incisura, gastric antrum, and pyloroplasty were normal. The duodenal bulb, 2nd part of the duodenum, area of the papilla and 3rd part of the duodenum was normal.

**Impression:** Benign-appearing esophageal stricture

Normal gastric body, incisura, antrum, and pyloroplasty

Normal duodenal bulb, 2nd part of duodenum, area of the papilla, and 3rd part of the duodenum

**Recommendation:** Discharge patient to home (ambulatory)

# CASE 10

# Access to central venous circulation

**Pre-operative Diagnosis:** Left breast cancer

**Post-operative Diagnosis:** Left breast cancer

**Procedures Performed:** Placement of subclavian Port-a-Cath

Fluoroscopic guidance for placement of the catheter

**Surgeon:** Dr. Optum

**Anesthesia:** General and approximately 14 mL of 0.25% Marcaine without epinephrine locally

Anesthesiologist, DD performed the general endotracheal anesthesia for the case while running two procedures concurrently (PS IV)

The surgeon placed an arterial catheter in the right radial artery at the beginning of the case.

**Anesthesia start time:** 8:00 A.M. **Anesthesia end time:** 9:05 A.M.

**Complications:** None known

**Estimated Blood Loss:** Minimal

**Indications for Procedure:** This is a very pleasant, 71-year-old female who was recently found to have left breast cancer with metastatic disease to her left axillary lymph nodes. The patient was seen by her oncologist who felt that she would benefit from chemotherapy. I was asked to place a venous access tonight so she could receive her chemotherapy. After a long discussion with her oncologist and internist about risks and benefits, it was decided to proceed with this surgery.

**Findings:** A right subclavian Port-a-Cath was placed under fluoroscopic guidance. The catheter was placed into the superior vena cava. It flushed easily. There was good blood return. It was flushed again. Post-operative chest x-ray showed good placement of the catheter with no evidence of pneumothorax or other problems.

**Description of Procedure:** The patient was taken to the operating room and placed on the table in a supine position. After adequate general anesthesia, the patient was properly positioned on the operating room table. Using a marking pen, the anatomic landmarks and the proposed site for the port and the catheter were marked. The operative field was then infiltrated with 14 mL of 0.25% Marcaine without epinephrine. Using a needle and syringe, the right subclavian vein was entered. A guidewire was passed through the needle down the superior vena cava and then down into the inferior vena cava. This was done to make absolutely certain I was in the venous circulation. A small incision was made at the needle site. Under fluoroscopic guidance, the dilator was passed over the guidewire. The dilator and introducer were then passed over the guidewire. The guidewire was removed. The dilator was removed leaving the introducer. The catheter, which had been previously cut and flushed with heparinized saline, was then passed through the introducer, into the superior vena cava. The peel-away introducer was removed. The catheter was aspirated, and dark venous blood was obtained. It was promptly positioned under fluoroscopic guidance. It was then sutured at the skin with a 3-0 Vicryl at approximately the 15 cm mark. It was clamped.

The subcutaneous pocket was then made. Great care was taken to make sure there was no evidence of any bleeding. The catheter was tunneled to the pocket. The catheter was then connected to the port and locked into place. The port was aspirated using a Huber needle. Dark venous blood returned. It was then flushed until clear. It was sutured to the pectoralis major fascia with three sutures of 3-0 silk. Both wounds were dry. They were closed with 3-0 Vicryl and 4-0 Monocryl. Dressings were applied. A postoperative chest x-ray showed good placement of the catheter with no evidence of pneumothorax.

The patient was then moved to the recovery room in stable condition.

CASE 11

# Cardiac catheterization

**Description**

A 49-year-old female presented to the emergency department (ED) with the sudden onset of retrosternal chest pain with radiation to her jaw and left arm.

**Chief complaint**

Chest pain with jaw and left arm radiation.

**History of present illness**

The patient described an episode of chest pain with arm and jaw radiation that occurred suddenly while she was working in her yard. The episode lasted approximately 15 minutes. She chewed and swallowed four ASA, with some resolution of the pain. However, she was still having pain intermittently. Her chest pain was accompanied by generalized weakness and shortness of breath.

**Review of systems**

The patient appears anxious and diaphoretic.

**Personal history**

Positive for hypothyroidism.

**Social history**

Denies smoking, ETOH use, illicit drug use. Very recently widowed (two months ago). She has two daughters, alive and well.

**Family history**

**Medications**

Synthroid 75 mcg. Multivitamin and calcium supplements daily.

**Allergies**

**NKA**

**Physical examination**

Thin female, alert and oriented. Appears anxious, somewhat dyspneic.

**Vital signs:** BP 140/86; Pulse 100; Respirations 24; O2 sat 100% on 2 liters/minute via nasal cannula; Temperature 37.2 degrees C.

**Course in the emergency department**

The patient was evaluated in the ED and worked up for myocardial ischemia. She underwent cardiac catheterization and was admitted to the cardiac care unit for monitoring and continued evaluation.

**Procedures**

A transthoracic echocardiogram (TTE) was performed. It demonstrated a regional wall motion abnormality in the apex of the left ventricle, which corroborated the suspicion of myocardial ischemia.

**Diagnostic studies**

Cardiac enzymes and cardiac markers somewhat elevated. Serial EKGs demonstrate ST-T changes, suggestive of myocardial ischemia.

**Treatment**

Cardiac monitoring was initiated. The patient was provided with nitroglycerin, simvastatin, and IV metoprolol. Supplemental oxygen was applied by nasal cannula at 2 liters. Morphine was given for pain. The pain dissipated and she was much more comfortable.

She underwent emergency left heart catheterization, which revealed Takotsubo cardiomyopathy.

**Anesthesia:** General endotracheal

Anesthesiologist, MM personally performed the general endotracheal anesthesia for the case with the help of two CRNAs (PS III)

The anesthesiologist placed a Swan Ganz catheter and performed a transesophageal echocardiogram (TEE) at the beginning of the case.

**Anesthesia start time:** 04:25 A.M. **Anesthesia end time:** 07:37 A.M.

The anesthesiologist accompanied the patient to the PACU after the end of the procedure performed in the operating room.

**Impression**

Possible acute coronary syndrome.

**Plan**

Admit patient to the cardiac care unit, cardiac MRI in the AM. Resume Synthroid.

# CASE 12

# Cardiac catheterization

**Description**

A 51-year-old male patient presented with a three-week history of worsening shortness of breath, fatigue, swelling in his legs, palpitations, and near syncope.

**Chief complaint**

The patient complained of difficulty breathing, swelling of his legs bilaterally, and palpitations that have become progressively worse.

**History of present illness**

The patient noticed a gradual onset of shortness of breath and fatigue a few months ago. In the past three weeks, those symptoms have worsened, and the patient now palpitations, leg edema, and has had a couple of episodes of near syncope.

**Review of systems**

**Vital signs:** BP 100/62; P 112: R20; Pulse oximetry 94%; Temp. 97.8.

**General:** Male patient; appears than stated age; weight appropriate for height.

**Past medical history**

Back injury with damage many years ago. Repair of a torn rotator cuff.

**Social history**

Patient lives with his wife. He is a surveyor and owns his own company. He has one grown son living out of state. Does not smoke; drinks socially. Denied of use of illegal substances.

**Family history**

Mother has hypertension, atrial fibrillation. Father has a history of CAD. Three siblings are alive and well.

**Medications**

PRN use of Skeleton and Motrin for recurrent back pain. Multivitamins.

**Allergies**

**NKA.**

**Physical examination**

**General:** Some cyanosis of lips and nail beds noted.

**HEENT:** Significant for engorgement of jugular veins.

**Heart:** Significant for a gallop and loud pulmonic valve component.

**Abdomen:** Ascites noted; normal BS.

**Extremities:** Edema of legs and ankles bilateral.

# CASE

**Diagnostic Studies:** Laboratory Studies ordered.

Electrolytes, BUN, creatinine, LFTs.

ANA, ESR.

Thyroid stimulating hormone (TSH).

HIV.

Arterial blood gases.

CBC.

B-type natriuretic (BNP).

**Diagnostic studies:** Other studies

Chest x-ray (done in the clinic): Significant for enlargement of right ventricle and enlargement of pulmonary arteries.

**EKG (done in clinics):** Suggestive of right ventricular hypertrophy.

Diagnostics tests ordered.

Doppler echocardiogram.

Ventilation-perfusion scan (V/Q scan).

Pulmonary function tests.

Will schedule right heart catheterization.

**Treatment**

Lasix and Cardizem.

**Impression**

Idiopathic primary pulmonary hypertension.

**Plan**

Admit patient to the telemetry unit in critical care. Will obtain results of the test as ordered, schedule heart catheterization in 105 minutes. Start the patient on Lasix and Cardizem for now. Consider anticoagulants, home O2 when discharged. Will base further treatment on the results of tests.

**Procedure:** Right heart catheterization including coronary angiography and ventriculography (not to include Swan-Ganz catheter)

**Anesthesia:** General endotracheal

Anesthesiologist, MM performed the general endotracheal anesthesia for the case personally (PS III)

**Anesthesia start time:** 08:00 A.M. **Anesthesia end time:** 10:50 A.M.

# CASE 13

## *Critical care*

**Admitted**: 8-3-XX **Discharged**: 8-4-XX

**Discharge Diagnosis**: ST elevation anteroseptal myocardial infarction, Hypertension, Chronic anemia

**Critical care time:** 2 hours

**Procedure:** Streptokinase infusion (PS IV)

This 76-year-old female was admitted to the hospital early in the morning with a complaint of chest pain, which began about two hours prior to admission. Cardiogram showed the presence of an anteroseptal myocardial injury pattern. The patient has known hypertension and chronic anemia. The patient was given streptokinase infusion via a peripheral vein percutaneous approach in the ED and was then sent to CCU for two hours. The patient initially did well but became unstable. The family asked that the patient is transferred to a larger facility. The patient was transferred to University Medical Center.

CASE 14

# Moderate (conscious) sedation

This 38-year-old female patient was admitted to evaluate the cause of uncontrollable abdominal discomfort. The patient has been experiencing intermittent dysphagia as well. The patient also has hypertension. The patient's abdominal discomfort was brought under control, and the next day the patient was sent to the GI lab for a procedure to determine the cause of the abdominal discomfort.

**Preoperative Diagnosis**: Intermittent dysphagia and upper abdominal discomfort. The patient had a history of peptic ulcer disease in the past.

**Postoperative Diagnosis**: Moderate duodenitis. Prepyloric ulcer and gastritis in the antrum. Hiatal hernia 5 centimeters.

**Operation**: Esophagogastroduodenoscopy

**Surgeon:** NN, MD

**Anesthesiologist:** MM, MD

**Anesthesia:** Moderate conscious sedation (MCS) with intravenous Versed 4 milligrams

Anesthesiologist personally performed the moderate conscious sedation for the case for an intraservice time of 27 minutes (PS III)

**Operation**: Esophagogastroduodenoscopy

Intravenous anesthesia administered as described above. Monitoring of sedation was assisted by an R.N. After the patient's throat was well-anesthetized, well-lubricated single channel Olympus gastroscope GIF100 was inserted, advanced without difficulty into the stomach, then into the duodenum. Duodenum 1st portion, moderate duodenitis. There is a narrow area, but the mucosa appears to be intact between the 1st and 2nd portions of the duodenum. 2nd portion of the duodenum is normal. This narrow area I couldn't visualize very well, probably because it is at the angulation. Mucosa, whatever portion I can see, appeared to be normal. This could be secondary to healed peptic ulcer disease. Antrum of the stomach, the patient has multiple superficial linear ulcerations consistent with a prepyloric ulcer. Lesser curvature, greater curvature, the fundus of the stomach were all within normal limits. The patient is noted to have 5-centimeter hiatal hernia. No evidence of any reflux esophagitis. The entire esophagus is within normal limits.

**Final Diagnosis:** Abdominal discomfort secondary to a prepyloric ulcer, antral gastritis, and moderate duodenitis; dysphagia-like symptoms might actually be gastroesophageal reflux from hiatal hernia rather than dysphagia; hypertension

# CASE 15

# *Open or surgical arthroscopy*

**Preoperative Diagnosis**: Displaced comminuted fracture of the lateral condyle, right elbow

**Postoperative Diagnosis**: Displaced comminuted fracture of the lateral condyle, right elbow

**Procedure:** Open reduction, internal fixation

**Anesthesia:** General endotracheal

**Anesthesiologist:** CRNA, FR, MD provided the anesthesia for the case without the help of or direction by an anesthesiologist (PS III)

**Anesthesia start time:** 8:05 A.M. **Anesthesia end time:** 10:59 A.M.

**Description:** The 55-year-old male patient, with malignant hypertension and type 1 diabetes mellitus, was anesthetized and prepped with Betadine, sterile drapes were applied, and the pneumatic tourniquet was inflated around the arm. An incision was made in the area of the lateral epicondyle through a Steri-Drape, and this was carried through subcutaneous tissue, and the fracture site was easily exposed. The inspection revealed the fragment to be rotated in two planes about 90 degrees. It was possible to manually reduce this quite easily, and the judicious manipulation resulted in an almost anatomic reduction. This was fixed with two pins driven across the humerus. These pins were cut off below skin level. The wound was closed with some plain catgut subcutaneously and 5-0 nylon in the skin. Dressings were applied to the patient and tourniquet released. A long arm cast was applied.

CASE 16

# Open or surgical arthroscopic/endoscopic

This 52-year-old male was brought to the same-day surgery area for treatment of an open fracture of the distal phalanx of his index finger on the left hand. The patient is right-handed and this injury occurred when the food-processing machine that he was operating at work tipped over and his hand got caught. He works in the local food factory here in town. The patient had open treatment performed to remove the fracture fragments without any internal or external fixation hardware used.

**Procedure:** Open treatment of fracture of the distal phalanx of the index finger of the left hand without any internal or external fixation devices

**Anesthesia:** General endotracheal

**Anesthesiologist:** HD, MD provided the anesthesia for the case while directing 5 CRNAs (PS II)

5 CRNAs, JJ, MD, FD, MD, KL, MD, NN, MD, and SD, MD under the direction of the anesthesiologist

There was emergency bleeding during the surgical case of 500 ml in total.

**Anesthesia start time:** 8:00 A.M. **Anesthesia end time:** 10:22 A.M.

CASE 17

# Direct coronary artery bypass graft

**Preoperative Diagnosis**: Severe coronary artery disease

**Postoperative Diagnosis**: Severe coronary artery disease

**Operative Procedure:** Cardiac bypass grafting

**Anesthesia:** General endotracheal

**Anesthesiologist:** AS, MD directed two CRNAs for the anesthesiology case (PS III)

Two CRNAs, MK, MD and HG, MD under the direction of the anesthesiologist

**Anesthesia start time:** 9:25 A.M. **Anesthesia end time:** 3:07 P.M.

**Procedure:** CABG x 4; saphenous vein graft to the obtuse marginal, diagonal artery and posterior descending artery; left internal mammary artery to the left anterior descending artery; cardiopulmonary bypass

**Details:** After obtaining adequate anesthesia, the 55-year old patient was prepped and draped. A primary median sternotomy incision was made, and the pericardium was opened. The left internal mammary artery was dissected as a pedicle using electrocautery and small hemoclips at the same time that the greater saphenous vein was harvested endoscopically from the left lower extremity. Cardiopulmonary bypass was instituted, and the patient was taken to a mild degree of hypothermia. The saphenous vein graft was placed end-to-end with the posterior descending artery, then a separate graft was placed to obtuse marginal and finally a separate graft to a diagonal artery. The left internal mammary artery was subsequently brought through a subthalamic tunnel and placed end-to-side with the left anterior descending coronary artery. Following completion of grafts, warm blood cardioplegia was administered, and the patient was weaned from cardiopulmonary bypass. The incision was closed, and the patient was taken to recovery in good condition.

CASE 18

# Cesarean delivery

**Post-operative diagnosis:** Complete placenta previa with hemorrhage; preterm labor with preterm delivery of twins; twin pregnancy; acute post-hemorrhagic anemia; anemia complicating childbirth

**Procedures:** Primary low cervical cesarean delivery of twins

Anesthesiologist, MM, MD personally provided the general endotracheal anesthesia for the case (PS III)

**Anesthesia start time:** 11:00 A.M. **Anesthesia end time:** 16:03 P.M.

The 25-year-old patient is admitted with vaginal bleeding. The patient has been admitted to labor and delivery several times during this pregnancy. The patient is 33 years old, gravida 1, para 0, and is at 33 weeks gestation. She has twin gestation (two placentae and two amniotic sacs) and complete placenta previa. Because of this last episode of bleeding, it was decided to keep the patient at bed rest in labor and delivery at the hospital so that, should any further excessive bleeding occur, she would be available for emergency cesarean delivery, if necessary. The intent was to keep her until she reached 36 weeks gestation, as recommended by the perinatologist in consultation. One day prior to reaching 36 weeks gestation, the patient had bright red bleeding. It was decided to go forward with a primary low cervical cesarean delivery for the complete placenta previa with hemorrhage. The patient delivered a 4 pound, 9 ounces viable female with Apgars of 8 and 9 at 16:01 p.m. Subsequently, she delivered a 4 pound, 15 ounces viable male with Apgars of 7 and 9 at 16:03 p.m. Intraoperative blood loss was approximately 1 liter. The patient was anemic due to acute blood loss prior to surgery. She had a good recovery, and her hemoglobin stabilized at 8.2. She was discharged home to follow-up in the office in 2 weeks for an incision check.

# CASE 19

# *Central venous circulation*

An 8-year-old male hemophiliac is admitted with acute blood loss anemia following uncontrolled bleeding. A peripherally inserted central venous catheter (PICC) without a subcutaneous port or pump is placed. He was given four units of packed red blood cells via the peripheral vein. While in the hospital he also received his regular preventive infusion of clotting factors.

Anesthesiologist MM, MD performed the general endotracheal anesthesia for the case while directing 2 CRNAs. JJ, MD, LK, MD (PS III)

The patient was in a prone position for the procedure. The anesthesia was complicated by utilization of controlled hypotension for 25 minutes.

**Anesthesia start time:** 9:00 A.M. **Anesthesia end time:** 9:57 A.M.

## CASE 20

# Integumentary system

**Operative Note**

**Preoperative Diagnosis:** Upper-outer quadrant breast lump

**Postoperative Diagnosis:** Right Breast Fibroadenoma

**Procedure:** Right Breast fibroadenoma excisional biopsy

Anesthesiologist, JF, MD personally provided the general endotracheal anesthesia for the case while directing 5 CRNAs, KL, MD, MN, MD, ND, MD, GG, MD. WR, MD (PS II)

A central venous pressure Swan-Ganz catheter was placed at the beginning of the case by the surgeon.

There was an emergency condition of emergency bleeding during the anesthesia for the case.

**Anesthesia start time:** 7:00 A.M. **Anesthesia end time:** 7:35 A.M.

The 35-year old patient was admitted, prepped, and taken to surgery. Following general anesthesia, the right breast was prepped and draped in sterile fashion. The mass was again palpated and found to be over 1.0 cm. in diameter. An incision was made at the 12 o'clock to 9 o'clock position. The incision was carried down through the skin and into the breast tissue. The mass was pushed in a medial fashion, grasped with a tenaculum, and excised in toto. It was sent immediately for histologic examination, which revealed it to be a fibroadenoma. Hemostasis was achieved with a combination of electrocautery and point ligation. It was decided to leave a drain in place. The subcutaneous tissues were closed with interrupted sutures of 4-0 chromic, and the skin was closed with 5-0 Vicryl. The drain was brought out through a separate incision. Steri-Strips were applied to secure the wounds. A bulky dressing was placed and secured with Elastoplast tape. Estimated blood loss was less than 500 cc under emergency bleeding during the case, and the patient tolerated the procedure well. The patient's postoperative course was uneventful. The patient was discharged home to see me at my office in follow-up in 10 days.

CASE 21

# Thoracotomy utilizing 1 lung ventilation

**Discharge Summary**

**Admitted**: 4-13-XX Discharged: 4-18-XX

**History**: This 45-year-old male was status post right nephrectomy two years ago for carcinoma of the kidney. He was admitted this time with a left lung mass and was found to have metastatic renal carcinoma to the lung.

**Hospital Course**: On 4/14, the patient underwent left thoracotomy with wedge excision of his left upper lobe mass. Postoperatively, the patient did well. The chest tube was removed on 4/17 and discharged on 4/18.

Anesthesiologist, LK, MD provided the monitored anesthesia care (MAC) service for the case while directing one CRNA, HG, MD (PS IV)

**Anesthesia start time:** 11:47 A.M. **Anesthesia end time:** 2:39 P.M.

CASE 22

# Moderate (conscious) sedation

**Ambulatory Setting**

**Endoscopy Report**

**Preoperative Diagnosis**: Rectal mass; Change in bowel habits

**Postoperative Diagnosis**: Rectal prolapse, rectal polyps, significant sigmoid diverticulosis with nonspecific colitis

**Procedure:** Colonoscopy performed to the level of the cecum, The 42-year-old patient was prepped in the usual fashion followed by placement in the left lateral decubitus position. I administered 3 mg of Versed. Monitoring of sedation was assisted by a trained R.N. Next, the Pentax Video Endoscope was passed through the rectal verge after a negative digital exam and advanced to the level of the cecum. The scope was then slowly retracted with a circular tip motion. There was mild nonspecific colitis noted. She did have significant sigmoid diverticulosis and several small polyps just inside the rectum, as well as a large prolapsing mass of mucosa approximately 5 cm inside the rectum. This appears to have prolapsed previously. Two of the small polyps were biopsied using the cold biopsy forceps and sent to pathology for the exam. The remainder of the exam was unremarkable. The patient tolerated the procedure well.

**Moderate conscious sedation for 25 minutes utilizing Versed was provided by the surgeon, JJ, MD as the anesthesiologist who was the same physician that performed the procedure**

**Pathology Report**: Clinical Information: Change in bowel habits. Colonoscopy performed. Gross exam: The specimen is labeled two polyps at 3 cm. Submitted are two fragments of tan tissue measuring tip to 0.3 cm in greatest dimension.

**Microscopic Exam**: Sections examined at multiple levels show two fragments of rectal mucosa in which the surfaces and subjacent crypts show no evidence of adenomatous or neoplastic changes.

**Diagnosis**: Rectum, biopsies at 3 cm rectal polyps.

# CASE 23

## *Sympathetic lumbar block*

**Post-operative diagnosis:** Phantom limb pain

A 55-year-old female patient with a right below-the-knee amputation and osteosarcoma of the fibula suffers from significant pain in the right lower limb where the right leg was before amputation. The patient has received chemotherapy for the osteosarcoma bone malignancy.

**Procedure:** Right lumbar sympathetic block

Injection of Marcaine and epinephrine into the L2 spinal space in hopes of providing relief for the pain

Anesthesiologist, DD, MD personally performed the right lumbar sympathetic nerve block (PS IV)

**Anesthesia start time:** 7:00 A.M. **Anesthesia end time:** 7:25 A.M.

# CASE 24

## Bone marrow aspiration

This 28-year-old patient with an abnormal blood test underwent bone marrow aspiration from the sternum. The area was cleaned with an antiseptic solution, and a local anesthetic was injected. The needle was inserted beneath the skin and rotated into the cortex and the sample taken. The needle was repositioned slightly, and a new syringe attached, and a second sample was obtained. These were sent to the laboratory for analysis. The results show acute lymphocytic leukemia (ALL).

**Post-operative diagnosis:** Acute lymphocytic leukemia

**Procedure:** Bone marrow aspiration from the sternum

Anesthesiologist, MM, MD provided the general endotracheal anesthesia for the case while directing 2 CRNAs (PS IV)

**CRNAs:** FF, MD, and JL, MD

**Anesthesia start time:** 7:50 A.M. **Anesthesia end time:** 9:17 A.M.

CASE 25

# Central venous circulation

The elderly 74-year-old male patient was seen in the same day surgery unit for insertion of a subclavian venous catheter for treatment of his prostate carcinoma.

**Post-operative diagnosis:** Prostate carcinoma

**Procedure:** Insertion of a percutaneous subclavian venous catheter

Anesthesiologist, KJ, MD personally provided the general endotracheal anesthesia for the case (PS IV)

**Anesthesia start time:** 9:47 A.M. **Anesthesia end time:** 10:42 A.M.

**Operative Report:** The patient's right upper chest was prepped and draped in the usual manner. General endotracheal anesthesia was performed. A percutaneous subclavian venous catheter was inserted and secured at the skin level with 4-0 nylon. A sterile dressing was applied. The catheter was irrigated with Heparin and the patient was sent to recovery.

# CASE 26

## *Integumentary system, muscles, nerves*

**Central Valley Hospital**

**1017 Rose Garden Ln.**

**Burley, ID 83768**

**PATIENT:** Smith, Jackie

**Age:** 66

**DATE OF SERVICE:** 01/01/20XX

Private Payer (Medicare rules for 65 years or older)

**PREOPERATIVE DIAGNOSIS:** Mass in the left upper chest overlying the head of the left clavicle.

**POSTOPERATIVE DIAGNOSIS:** Mass in the left upper chest overlying the head of the left clavicle, probable lymph node.

**PROCEDURE PERFORMED:** Excision of mass measuring about 1 x 1.5 cm.

**SURGEON:** John Andrews, MD

**ASSISTANT:** John Smith, RN

**ANESTHESIOLOGIST:** John Thompson, MD personally medically directed one CRNA for the case. JT, MD placed a non-tunneled central venous catheter into the right internal jugular vein at the beginning of the case (PS III)

**CRNA:** MM, CRNA

**ANESTHESIA:** Mask general endotracheal.

**Anesthesia start time:** 7:00 A.M. **Anesthesia end time:** 8:55 A.M.

**ESTIMATED BLOOD LOSS:** Negligible.

**PROCEDURE PERFORMED:** The 55-year-old patient was taken to the operative suite and following induction of general anesthesia, was sterilely prepped and draped in routine fashion. We had previously demarcated the area in the surgical holding area. 0.5% Marcaine with epinephrine was injected along our proposed line of incision around the mass. An incision was then made overlying the mass. This was carried into the subcutaneous tissues. At this point, blunt dissection was used to dissect out the mass. This was grasped with pickups and dissected out with electrocautery and blunt dissection. This was passed off the field to be sent to pathology. The subcutaneous and subcuticular tissue was approximated with 3-0 Vicryl followed by Dermabond. The patient was transferred to the recovery room in apparent satisfactory condition.

**GROSS PATHOLOGY:** This is a very pleasant 67-year-old female who presents with a mass overlying her left clavicular head. It was quite firm to palpate somewhat and moveable. I thought initially it was a deep subcutaneous cyst. This had an appearance of a lymph node and measured about 1 x 1.5 cm in size. No other gross pathology was noted.

Electronically signed by John Andrews, MD.

**Central Valley Hospital**

**Pathology Center**

**1017 Rose Garden Ln.**

**Burley, ID 83768**

**PATIENT:** Smith, Jackie

**Age:** 67

**DATE OF SERVICE:** 01/01/20XX

**PATHOLOGY REPORT**

**DIAGNOSIS:** Benign neoplasm of peripheral nerves and autonomic nervous system of the thorax

**COMMENTS:** The lesion represents an encapsulated, well-circumscribed lesion comprised of spindle cells containing elongated, wavy nuclei and eosinophilic cytoplasm which are prominent separated by ground substance. Solid areas are present, but the cell of origin is not clear on H&E stains. Mild nuclear atypia is present, but mitotic activity is not seen. A small battery of immunostains was performed and includes S-100, desmin, smooth muscle actin, smooth muscle myosin, and CD34. The S-100 is strongly positive and the CD34 demonstrates blush positivity. The desmin, smooth muscle actin, and smooth muscle myosin are all negative. This immunostain pattern would support the diagnosis of a benign nerve/nerve sheath tumor, and neurofibroma is favored, although benign neuro thecoma cannot be totally excluded. Correlation is suggested.

**SPECIMENS:** Left chest mass.

**GROSS DESCRIPTION:** Submitted in formalin and labeled "left chest mass" is a discoid shaped fragment of rubbery tan tissue measuring 1.0 x 1.0 x 0.6 cm. The surface is smooth and a small fragment of attached fat is identified. Section reveals a solid structure containing a semi-translucent light yellowish-tan cut surface. Entirely submitted in a single cassette.

**MICROSCOPIC DESCRIPTION:** All stains and controls are adequate.

Electronically signed by John Kramer, MD.

# CASE 27

# *Non-invasive or radiation therapy*

**RADIOLOGY REPORT**

**Valley Hospital**

**PATIENT:** Hedy Smith

**AGE:** 73

**DATE OF EXAM:** 1/1/20XX

Private Payer (Medicare rules for 65 or older) **Professional and technical modifiers are not required.**

The patient is a Medicare-insured patient.

**REFERRING PHYSICIAN(S):** Robert Thompson M.D.

**Anesthesiologist:** JJ, MD personally provided the monitored anesthesia care (MAC) service for the case (PS III)

**Procedure start time:** 7:57 A.M. **Procedure end time:** 8:42 A.M.

**PROCEDURE:** MRI BRAIN WITHOUT CONTRAST

**COMPARISON:** CT study dated 08/30/20XX.

**INDICATIONS:** Encephalopathy. A question of a pineal cyst.

**TECHNIQUE:** Sagittal FLAIR; axial T1, FLAIR, fast spin echo T2, and diffuse weighted images were obtained.

**FINDINGS:** The ventricles are normal size for age. There is no shift. No abnormal extra-axial fluid collections. On the T2 weighted images, there are some scattered areas of the bright signal in the white matter tracts superiorly. These are probably old gliosis changes. No signs of any extra-axial fluid collections. No new masses are seen. There are no signs of any expanding mass lesions in the pineal region. There is no abnormal signal change to suggest any new ischemia or new hemorrhage.

**CONCLUSION:**

1. Encephalopathy.

Electronically signed by TECHNICIAN 1/1/20XX

# CASE 28

## Non-invasive imaging or radiation therapy

**RADIOLOGY REPORT**

**Valley Hospital**

**PATIENT:** Cedric Jones **SEX:** Male

**AGE:** 50

**DOS:** 1/1/20XX

Private Payer (Medicare rules for 65 or older) **Professional and technical modifiers are not required.**

Anesthesiologist, KL, MD medically directed 4 CRNAs while providing the general endotracheal anesthesia for the case (PS III)

A surgeon placed a non-tunneled central venous catheter in the right internal jugular vein patient at the beginning of the case

CRNAs GG, MD, JM, MD, MM, MD, FG, MD

**Anesthesia start time:** 9:00 A.M.

**Anesthesia end time:** 9:55 A.M. which ended while the anesthesiologist and a CRNA were continuing medication administration at the end of anesthesia for the case

**PROCEDURE:** ABDOMEN CT WITH CONTRAST

**COMPARISON:** 10/31/20XX.

**INDICATIONS:** Abdominal pain.

**TECHNIQUE:** A volumetric acquisition was performed at 0.5 mm with multi-planar reformation. The study was performed with oral contrast and during the intravenous infusion of 100 ccs of Omnipaque-350.

**FINDINGS:**

**LOWER CHEST:** There is 5 mm ground-glass nodular density in the right lower lobe, Series 4 Image 6. This is better visualized on the current study as the dependent atelectasis seen in the lung bases on the previous study has resolved. There is some linear atelectasis in the left upper lobe.

**LIVER/BILIARY:** There is a heterogeneous area of decreased attenuation in the posterior segment of the right lobe of the liver, Series 3 Image 26, measuring 2.1 x 1.5 cm. This is incompletely characterized by this single-phase contrast-enhanced study. This does appear to cause some slight contour deformity involving the posterior right lobe of the liver. This was present previously and allowing for slight differences in the scan plane and the phase of contrast, this is probably not significantly changed. No other focal liver lesions are identified.

**PANCREAS:** Normal.

**SPLEEN:** Normal.

**KIDNEYS:** Normal.

**ADRENALS:** Normal.

**AORTA/VASCULAR:** Normal.

**RETROPERITONEUM:** Normal.

**BOWEL/MESENTERY:** Normal. A normal appendix is visualized.

**ABDOMINAL WALL:** There is diastasis of the rectus abdominis muscles anteriorly with herniation of omental fat and small bowel into the diastatic defect. There appear to be some surgical changes, presumably related to previous hernia repair.

**BONES:** Normal for age.

**OTHER:** Negative.

**CONCLUSION:**

1. Diastasis of the rectus abdominis muscles with herniation of small bowel and fat through the diastatic defect. This is wide-necked, and there is no evidence of bowel obstruction. There are postsurgical changes of the anterior abdominal wall, presumably related to previous hernia repair.
2. The liver lesion represents a benign hepatic hemangioma. Low attenuation lesion in the posterior segment of the right lobe of the liver, which is mildly contour-deforming. There is also a 5 mm ground-glass nodular density in the right lower lobe of the lung. These are not significantly changed when compared to the prior study allowing for some differences in technique. Consider follow-up to document stability, particularly of the lung nodule.

Electronically signed by TECHNICIAN 1/1/20XX

CASE 29

# Diagnosis or therapeutic nerve blocks and injections

**John Andrews, MD**

**Surgery Center**

**1017 Rose Garden Ln.**

**Burley, ID 83768**

**PATIENT:** Britney Smith

**SEX:** Female

**AGE:** 76

Medicare-insured

**DATE OF SERVICE:** 01/01/20XX

**PREOPERATIVE DIAGNOSIS:** Recurrent painful Morton's neuroma third intermetatarsal space, left foot.

**POSTOPERATIVE DIAGNOSIS:** Recurrent painful Morton's neuroma third intermetatarsal space, left foot.

**PROCEDURE PERFORMED:** Radiofrequency ablation of third intermetatarsal space Morton's neuroma, left foot.

**SURGEON:** John Andrews, MD

**CRNA:** DD, MD provided the anesthesia for the case without the help of a directing anesthesiologist (PS III)

The anesthesia was complicated by utilization of controlled hypotension.

**Anesthesia start time:** 11:00 A.M. **Anesthesia end time:** 11:47 A.M.

**ANESTHESIA:** General inhalation anesthesia.

**DESCRIPTION OF PROCEDURE:** The patient was brought to the OR and placed on the operating table in the supine position. General inhalation anesthesia was administered per anesthesia services. The left foot was then prepped and draped in the usual and customary aseptic fashion. No tourniquet was applied. Utilizing intraoperative imaging, the right radiofrequency ablation cannula and needle was inserted and determined to be placed sufficiently. The procedure was started at the distal aspect of the third intermetatarsal space with three more applications working proximally one-half to three-quarters of an inch proximal with each application. Each application was initiated with sensory testing followed by muscle testing of the RF equipment. This was found to be negative. The radiofrequency was ramped up to temperature as determined by the equipment. It was held in place for approximately 60 seconds at each site. This being applied 4 times with sequential imaging to determine satisfactory placement, the procedure was completed. The area was then locally anesthetized with 0.5% Marcaine plain proximal to the surgical site. Band-Aids were applied to the needle puncture sites.

The patient was transported to the recovery room per gurney in apparent satisfactory condition. There were no complications to the anesthesia or the procedure.

Electronically signed by John Andrews, MD. 1/1/20XX

**John Andrews, MD**

**Surgery Center**

**1017 Rose Garden Ln.**

**Burley, ID 83768**

**PATIENT:** Britney Smith

**AGE:** 76

**DATE OF SERVICE:** 01/01/20XX

**CHIEF COMPLAINT:** Left foot pain.

**HISTORY OF PRESENT ILLNESS:** Patient is here with a complaint of neuroma pain in her left foot between the 3rd and 4thy. She states that she has had it removed several years ago and is now back causing her pain.

**PHYSICAL EXAMINATION:**

**VITAL SIGNS:** Weigh 147, height 5'3", BP 151/94, HR 89.

**DIAGNOSTIC IMAGING:** Foot 3V WB, left, x-ray; AP, LMO, Lat.

**MEDICATIONS:** Mobic, Lipitor, aspirin 81, Fosamax, Ranitidine.

**SOCIAL HISTORY:** Neurectomy.

**FAMILY HISTORY:** Father: Deceased. Mother: Deceased.

**SOCIAL HISTORY:** No smoking. Some alcohol.

**ALLERGIES:** AMOXICILLIN, GEOCILLIN, PENICILLIN, SULFA, VERAPAMIL, CECLOR.

REVIEW OF SYSTEMS:

**CARDIOLOGY:** Chest pain no. Congestive heart failure no. Heart attack no. Hypertension no. Murmurs no. Pacemaker no. Palpitations no.

**CONSTITUTIONAL:** Cold limbs and feet yes. Weight gain no. Weight loss no.

**DERMATOLOGY:** Ecchymosis no. Lumps no. Rash no. Skin cancer no.

**ENDOCRINOLOGY:** Excessive sweating no. Excessive thirst no.

**GASTROENTEROLOGY:** Abdominal pain no. Heartburn yes.

**HEMATOLOGY/LYMPH:** Abnormal bleeding no. Abnormal bruising no. Fevers no. Swollen glands no.

**MUSCULOSKELETAL:** Fracture no. Joint pain no. Joint stiffness no. Sprains/strains no.

**NEUROLOGY:** Gait difficulties no. Headache no. Seizures no. Tremor no. Weakness no.

**PSYCHOLOGY:** Anxiety no. Depression no. Panic attacks no.

**RESPIRATORY:** Nasal stuffiness no. Problems with anesthesia no. Shortness of breath no. Wheezing no.

Electronically signed by John Andrews, MD. 1/1/20XX

# CASE 30

# *Open or arthroscopic procedures*

Central Valley Surgical Hospital
1017 Rose Garden Ln.
Burley, ID 83768

**PATIENT:** Junior Smith

**SEX:** Male

**AGE:** 49

**DATE OF SERVICE:** 01/01/20XX

**PREOPERATIVE DIAGNOSIS:**

1. Torn medial meniscus, right knee.
2. Synovitis, right knee.
3. Chondromalacia of the medial femoral condyle, right knee.

**POSTOPERATIVE DIAGNOSIS:**

1. Torn Posterior horn medial meniscus, right knee.
2. Synovitis, right knee.
3. Chondromalacia of the medial femoral condyle, right knee.

**PROCEDURE PERFORMED:** Diagnostic and operative arthroscopy, right knee.

a. Partial medial meniscectomy,
b. Extensive synovectomy tricompartmental,
c. Chondroplasty of the medial femoral condyle,

**SURGEON:** John Andrews, MD

**ASSISTANT:** John Thompson, MD

**ANESTHESIOLOGIST:** John Smith, MD personally provided the general endotracheal anesthesia for the case while directing 2 CRNAs (PS III)

**Anesthesia start time:** 6:50 A.M. **Anesthesia end time:** 10:39 A.M.

**ESTIMATED BLOOD LOSS:** Minimal.

**TOURNIQUET TIME:** None.

**COMPLICATIONS:** None.

**INDICATIONS:** The patient is a 49-year-old white male well known to me as I have previously operated on his left knee. He has had a good outcome there and because of continued troubles with the right knee, he sought out advice and care for issues there. MRI at the diagnostic center revealed degenerative arthropathy and joint effusion, Baker's cyst which appears to be ruptured and findings of a subtle oblique undersurface tear of the posterior horn of the medial meniscus, soft tissue edema within the popliteal fossa and some osteochondral lesions seen in the medial femoral condyle. Treatment options were discussed and reviewed with the patient and he wished the above and informed consents obtained. The nature of the condition, inherent risks, complications, options and benefits associated with the procedure have been discussed and reviewed with the patient in detail and informed consent obtained.

**DESCRIPTION OF PROCEDURE:** The patient was taken to the operating room, put on the operative stretcher and placed on the operating table in the supine position. Under IV sedation the patient was orally intubated by Dr. Smith and general anesthetic administered.

A tourniquet was placed about the right mid-thigh and secured in place. The leg holding device was secured immediate distal to it and to the table in standard fashion. The anterior aspect of the right knee had been shaved. The entire right lower extremity distal to the leg holder was sterilely scrubbed, prepped and draped with sterile linens in the usual sterile orthopedic fashion.

The inferior pole of the patella and the medial and lateral border of the infrapatellar tendon were marked with a sterile skin marker. A #11 blade knife handle was used to make two stab like portal incisions first being just inferior and lateral to the junction of the inferior pole of the patella and lateral border of the infrapatellar tendon and the second portal incision was made just medial to the junction of the inferior pole of the patella and the medial border of the infrapatellar tendon. Through the lateral portal, the blunt arthroscopic cannula and trocar were inserted. The knee was brought up into full extension and both were passed traumatically through the patellofemoral interval and suprapatellar pouch. The trocar was removed and the arthroscope was placed in through the cannula and secured in place. The arthroscopic pump was connected to it and turned on and the joint distended. The arthroscope was withdrawn slowly and the inferior aspect of the patella appeared appropriate and no significant chondromalacia problems identified. The blunt probe was placed in through the portal and heavy hypertrophic thickened synovium shrouded the patellofemoral and medial and lateral compartment. A 4.0 side cutting synovial shaver was used to perform an extensive tricompartmental synovectomy. The VAPR wand from Mitek was used to coag the bleeders within the synovium. The knee was brought back down into flexion and valgus held by the assistant. Blunt probing of the medial compartment revealed some chondromalacia of the medial meniscus showed some undersurface tears in the posterior side that were displaceable medially with the blunt probe. Basket forceps of various sizes, shapes, and inclinations was used to perform a partial medial meniscectomy. The 4.0 side cutting synovial shaver was used to resect the meniscal trimmings and remnants. The remainder of the meniscus appeared intact and firm and in good repair. Slight contouring of the remaining posterior horn of the medial meniscus was carried out with the synovial shaver. The anterior and posterior cruciate ligaments were intact on visualization and blunt probing and no evidence of laxity or acute or chronic tears on drawer testing. The knee was placed in a figure of four posture held by the assistant. Blunt probing of the lateral femoral condyle and lateral tibial plateau and lateral meniscus showed the compartment to be relatively pristine. There was no evidence of acute articular cartilage defect. Appropriate patellofemoral tracking was noted on arthroscopic visualization. The lateral recess was checked and no other pathology identified. The back of the knee was percussed as the arthroscope was advanced into the suprapatellar pouch and the side cutting synovial shaver was allowed to turn in the suprapatellar pouch as well through the medial portal and any shaving or trimming remnants were evacuated by this technique and the VAPR wand again was used to obtain good hemostasis of bleeders within the synovium. At this point, all pathology within the knee was thought to be addressed and all instrumentation removed from the knee. The knee was injected with 0.25% Marcaine plain and lidocaine 1% plain. The portal incisions were closed with 4-0 nylon interrupted horizontal mattress stitch x1 for each incision site and covered with Xeroform, 4 x 4s, ABDs and 6 inch Ace wrap applied.

The patient tolerated the procedure well. There were no complications encountered intraoperatively. All sponge and needle counts were correct.

Electronically signed by John Andrews, MD. 1/1/20XX

# CASE 31

## *Vaginal*

**Women's Health Care**

**Central Valley Hospital**

**PATIENT:** Debra Smith

**SEX:** Female

**AGE:** 28

**Date of Service:** 1/1/20XX

Private Payer (Medicare rule for 65 or older)

**Chief Complaint:** Recurrent abnormal Pap smears and dysplasia. History of Present Illness: The Ne patient is seen for Dr. Kramer for recurrent abnormal Pap smears. Her history began in 20xx, at which time she had abnormal Pap smear. She then underwent cryotherapy for grade 2 dysplasia. She had a repeat colposcopy due to recurrent abnormal Pap smears in 2007. She had an ASCUS of negative HPV at one point, but then did have grade dysplasia present following a low-grade SIL Pap. She underwent LEEP in March of 20xx and showed grade 1-2 dysplasia with negative margins, endocervical and ectocervical. She then had a low-grade SIL Pap in September 20xx and had a biopsy showing focal atypia consistent with HPV effect. In January of 2009, ASCUS was positive HPV. In May, again, an ASCUS with positive HPV. She underwent colposcopic directed biopsy showing grade 1 dysplasia on the ectocervix; on 1 biopsy koilocytosis suggestive of HPV effect, on another ectocervical biopsy, and endocervical curettage was negative and did obtain tissue. Most recently in November, she had a Pap smear showing ASCUS positive HPV and is here today for a consultation. She has had no intramenstrual bleeding. She is on Ocella for oral contraceptives and this has helped with her premenstrual pain. She is sexually active, has had no infections and has had normal periods.GYN History; Gravida 0, menarche at 11-12, 28-day cycles, the above mentioned Pap smear History

**Past Medical History:** Asthma

**Past Surgical History:** Cryotherapy and LEEP

**Family History:** No breast, ovary, uterine, or colon cancer

**Allergies:** No known drug allergies.

**Medications:** Ocella, allergy pills and as needed inhaler.

**Social History:** No tobacco use, occasional alcohol use.

**Physical Exam:**

**Vital Signs:** Ht 5 ft. 1, wt. 182, Bp 133/72, temp 99.1, pulse 90, saturation 98%.

**General:** Well developed, well-nourished woman in no apparent distress.**Abdomen:** Soft, non-tender, no rebound, guarding, fluid wave, or distention. No hepatosplenomegaly

**Extremities:** Non-tender, no edema Pelvic: Normal external genitalia including Bartholin's, urethra, and Skenes. Speculum shows normal vaginal vault, bladder based posterior vagina, and cervix. The cervix is status post LEEP but has good normal appearing architecture and good length of the cervix within the vaginal vault. After informed consent was obtained and an hCG was negative, the cervix was evaluated with colposcopy. Acetic acid was applied. There were no nonstaining areas, the entire vagina was visualized. Lugol's was also applied and the entire vagina and cervix was visualized. A 1 mm nonstaining area was noted. Bimanual exam reveals no masses. No cul-de-sac nodularity. The cervical length appears at least 4-5 cm.

Anesthesiologist, JK, MD provided the general endotracheal anesthesia for the case (PS III)

**Anesthesia start time:** 7:00 A.M. **Anesthesia end time:** 7:55 A.M.

**Assessment and Plan:** A patient gravida 0 with a history of grade 2 dysplasia treated by LEEP and has had prior cryotherapy. She has had remarkable retention of her normal anatomy, otherwise. I see no evidence of high-grade dysplasia and may see a 1 mm focus of medium changes. I have recommended that she continue to observe and we have discussed the difficulties observing the canal, but she did have a negative biopsy in June and/or July. Therefore, I have recommended a follow-up Pap smear in 6 months' time with Dr. Kramer, should this be normal, a follow-up Pap in 6 months time from then. Should this show a high-grade change then I would recommend a repeat evaluation given the prior grade 2 dysplasia and the possibility of missing other diseases in the canal. Should show ASCUS, then I would repeat colposcopy and Pap in 1 year from now. The patient is in agreement with this plan. We will let Dr. Brown of these recommendations as well.

Electronically Signed by John Andrews MD 1/1/20XX

# CASE 32

## *Vaginal*

**John Andrews, MD**

**Women's Cancer Center**

**1017 Rose Garden Ln.**

**Burley, ID 83768**

**PATIENT:** Sarah Smith

**SEX:** Female

**AGE:** 42

**DATE OF SERVICE:** 01/01/20XX

Private Payer (Medicare rules for 65 or older)

**CHIEF COMPLAINT:** Severe Vulvar dysplasia.

**HISTORY OF PRESENT ILLNESS:** The new patient is a 42-year-old seen for vulvar dysplasia. She underwent a biopsy revealing grade 3 dysplasia. Her history is complicated, both in her general medical history, as well as her gynecologic history. She reports having LEEP procedure and cold knife cone in 2006, results of which I do not have today. She believes that she did have an abnormal Pap and that is what brought her back in to see her doctor. She reports a colposcopy performed in early January was negative, but vulvar lesions were biopsied. She reports a colposcopy performed in early January was negative, but vulvar lesions were biopsied. She reports that she has had itching and burning on her vulva for a number of months. Initially, these were felt to be a nonneoplastic process that was more like sebaceous cysts and had been recommended to just help extrude the cystic contents, but these bumps continued. They have now kind of coalesced in a posterior fourchette at the site of what has now been biopsied. She reports that in the last 2 weeks, she has also had bleeding from her rectum and she does not believe it is associated particularly with constipated stools. She has occasional nausea and vomiting but no fever or chills.

Her history medically is complicated by autoimmune disease and specifically, she has had interstitial fibrosis, polymyositis, and rheumatoid arthritis. She is seen and managed now for her rheumatoid arthritis. She reports having received chemotherapy one and a half years ago for this. She has polymyositis associated with interstitial lung disease. She does not have pulmonary fibrosis. She was hospitalized in 01/20XX for acute respiratory failure and was in the intensive care unit from 01/04/20XX through 01/16/20XX. There was felt to be a viral syndrome on top of her baseline pulmonary disease. She reports that her pulmonary function has greatly improved and this was a superimposed acute process. She is now following with Dr. Thompson, who has seen her in 01/20XX. Pulmonary function tests have been now obtained as an outpatient to continue her forward. Her rectal bleeding has not yet been addressed.

**REVIEW OF SYSTEMS:** Otherwise negative.

**GYNECOLOGIC HISTORY:** Gravida 5, para 3-0-2-3 with 2 vaginal deliveries, 1 cesarean section. Menarche at 12. Her last period was 4 years ago. She has had no bleeding since her chemo.

**PAST MEDICAL HISTORY:** Polymyositis and interstitial lung disease.

**PAST SURGICAL HISTORY:** She reports lung surgery, vein ligation, breast augmentation, the right eye was removed possibly for tumor or trauma when she was 3, cesarean section x1.

**FAMILY HISTORY:** Maternal aunt with ovarian cancer. Maternal aunt, a second one, with ovarian cancer, a maternal aunt with some pelvic cancer.

**ALLERGIES:** SULFA and possibly LATEX.

MEDICATIONS:

1. Gabapentin.
2. Imuran 100 mg b.i.d.
3. Folic acid.
4. Dapsone.
5. Wellbutrin b.i.d.
6. Prozac.
7. Potassium.
8. Lortab 1 tab b.i.d.
9. Diclofenac b.i.d.
10. Multivitamin.
11. Calcium

**SOCIAL HISTORY:** No tobacco use, occasional alcohol use. The patient has a long term partner and previously married.

**PHYSICAL EXAMINATION: VITAL SIGNS:** Height is 5 feet 8 inches, weight 127, blood pressure 134/78, temperature 98.2, pulse 118 with saturation 91%.

**GENERAL:** Well-developed woman in no apparent distress.

**NECK:** There is no lymphadenopathy.

**LUNGS:** Clear to auscultation bilaterally.

**HEART:** Regular rate and rhythm with slight tachycardia.

**LYMPHATICS:** Neck and groin negative.**SKIN:** Normal throughout my examination.

**NEUROLOGIC:** Oriented to time, person and place. Normal affect.**PELVIC:** Normal external genitalia including Bartholin's, urethra, and Skenes. Grossly, there are multiple 2-3 mm raised lesions on the labia majora to the left and right leg folds an on to the anterior surface or mons. There is a gross lesion at the posterior fourchette extending in a U-shaped fashion approximately 3 cm in each direction, consistent with grade 3 dysplasia. A colposcopic examination was performed. There are no other acetowhite changes, however, the midline posterior fourchette in a U-shaped area of acetowhite consistent with grade 2 dysplasia. There is certainly some heterogeneity across the surface. Speculum exam shows normal vaginal vault, normal-appearing cervix. Colposcopy was also performed of the cervix and vagina due to the recent abnormal Pap. I see no known staining areas. Bimanual exam reveals no masses, smooth cul-de-sac. The cervix is not enlarged, no parametrial disease.

2 CRNAs, KK, CRNA, LL, CRNA performed the monitored anesthesia care for the case without the direction of an anesthesiologist (PS III)

**Anesthesia start time:** 4:45 P.M. **Anesthesia end time:** 6:02 P.M.

**Complications:** The anesthesia was complicated by emergency bleeding of 20 mL during the colposcopy of the cervix and vagina.

**RECTAL:** Not performed due to the patient's discomfort, but is at this point in the presence of examination.

**ASSESSMENT AND PLAN:** A 42-year-old with multiple medical problems, immunosuppression and now grade 3 dysplasia. I have discussed with the patient that this is HPV related and that 50-80% sexually active adults have been exposed across their lifetime in the patient with immunosuppressant drugs necessary for other diseases. These processes can be frequent and recurrent. I have recommended resection and discussed both resection and laser options. I do believe it will have a good cosmetic result and given the heterogeneity of the lesion, I would like to make sure there is no micro invasion or invasion present. The smaller lesions, more consistent with mild dysplasia, will be lasered. Risk of infection and bleeding were discussed. She is not on prednisone and will not need stress dose steroids. Two important things prior to surgery; one would be to ascertain her fitness for surgery whether we need to pursue spinal as opposed to intubation, as well as a workup of the rectal bleeding. I did not perform a rectal exam, as she is very uncomfortable at that point, but she does need to have a rectal evaluation and ideally with direct visualization. I have referred her to a colorectal surgeon and the instance that intraluminal disease requiring treatment may be required, a colonoscopy, hopefully, will be able to be performed, prior to pursuing her vulvar resection. The patient expresses an understanding of these processes and we will set a date pending her GI evaluation.

Electronically signed by John Andrews, MD. 1/1/20XX

**John Andrews, MD**

**Women's Cancer Center**

**1017 Rose Garden Ln.**

**Burley, ID 83768**

**DATE:** 01/01/20XX

**John, Thompson, MD**

**1234 E 4567 South, Suite 1A**

**Burley, ID 83768**

**RE:** Smith, Sarah

Dear Dr. Thompson,

I am writing to you regarding Sarah Smith, who as you know, is a complicated 42-year-old woman with vulvar dysplasia. I had the pleasure of meeting her on 01/01/20XX. Please see my enclosed dictation. In summary, I have recommended a combination of excision and laser. Prior to scheduling that, she hopefully will be obtaining a colonoscopic evaluation for new onset of rectal bleeding. I will certainly keep you updated as to our findings and progress. I very much appreciated the opportunity to become involved in this delightful lady's care.

Warmest regards,

John Andrews, MD 1/1/20XX

# CASE 33

# *Vaginal*

**John Andrews, MD**

**Women's Cancer Center**

**1017 Rose Garden Ln.**

**Burley, ID 83768**

**PATIENT:** Amanda Smith

**AGE:** 46

**DATE OF SERVICE:** 01/01/20XX

**Medicare Payer**

**CHIEF COMPLAINT:** Adnexal mass.

**HISTORY OF PRESENT ILLNESS:** The patient is a 46-year-old gravida 2, para 2, seen in consultation for an adnexal mass. The patient presented for an annual examination. At that time, her doctor felt an adnexal mass. An ultrasound was obtained. This revealed a cyst of 11.5 x 8.9 cm, arising from the right ovary, possible hemorrhagic or cystic neoplasm. The left ovary was normal in configuration. The uterus was measured 10 x 5.7 x 6.4 with a stripe of 7 mm. A 2.5 cm myoma in the fundal anterior portion was noted. No free fluid was mentioned. A CA-125 was obtained, which was 11. Other blood work demonstrated hematocrit 39.1, white count 5.4, normal BUN, creatinine and liver function tests normal, TSH. She also reports a longstanding history of rectocele, which she is not felt to be warranting intervention. She notes that she has to splint to help stool come out. She has also had a change in her periods over the last several months. She has a 3-month episode of amenorrhea followed by a very heavy period in May, and she has had some spotting since then. She has had some pressure and swelling in her rectum over the last several months and difficulty emptying her bowels. No nausea, vomiting, fever or chills, or blood in her stools.

**REVIEW OF SYSTEMS:** Otherwise negative on 14-point review.

**GYNECOLOGIC HISTORY:** Gravida 2, para 2 with 2 vaginal deliveries. Menarche at 15.

**PAST MEDICAL HISTORY:** Fibromyalgia, irritable bowel syndrome, GE reflux disease, herniated disk at L4-5.

**PAST SURGICAL HISTORY:** Left shoulder, right foot, and tonsils.

**SCREENING HISTORY:** Mammogram, 01/20XX, negative. Colonoscopy 6-7 years ago. Last Pap smear 01/20XX, which was normal.

**FAMILY HISTORY:** Father with small intestine cancer.

**ALLERGIES:** None.

**MEDICATIONS:** None.

**SOCIAL HISTORY:** No tobacco or alcohol use.

**PHYSICAL EXAMINATION:**

**VITAL SIGNS:** Height is 5 feet 7 inches, weight 180, blood pressure 115/62, temperature 98.9 degrees, pulse 85, saturation 99%.

**GENERAL:** Well-developed, well-nourished woman in no apparent distress.

**NECK:** There is no lymphadenopathy.

**LUNGS:** Clear to auscultation bilaterally.

**HEART:** Regular rate and rhythm without murmurs, rubs or gallops.

**LYMPHATICS:** Neck and groin negative.

**SKIN:** Normal throughout my examination.

**NEUROLOGIC:** Oriented to time, person and place. Normal affect.

**ABDOMEN:** Soft and nontender. There is a mass arising from the pelvis to the umbilicus. It is mobile. There is no rebound, guarding, fluid wave, or distention. No hepatosplenomegaly.

**EXTREMITIES:** Nontender, no edema.

**PELVIC:** Normal external genitalia, including Bartholin's, urethra, and Skenes. Speculum shows normal vaginal vault, bladder base, posterior vagina, and cervix. Bimanual exam reveals a mass arising from the mid pelvis to the umbilicus. There is no cul-de-sac nodularity. The uterus appears to move separately from this. There is no rectal mucosal abnormality.

**PROCEDURE:** After informed consent was obtained due to the patient's irregular bleeding, an endometrial biopsy was performed. The hCG was checked and found to be negative. The cervix was then cleansed with Betadine x3 and an endometrial sampler passed to 8 cm. Adequate tissue was obtained. The patient tolerated the procedure well.

Anesthesiologist, GN, MD performed the general endotracheal anesthesia for the case while medically directing one CRNA (PS III)

Anesthesiologist placed an arterial catheter in the right radial artery at the beginning of the case.

**Anesthesia start time:** 6:50 A.M. **Anesthesia end time:** 7:47 A.M.

**ASSESSMENT AND PLAN:** A 46-year-old with an adnexal mass. I have reviewed the ultrasound images personally and these appear to be mostly cystic with some thickening of the wall, but no clear nodularity. CA-125 is normal. I do favor a benign etiology, likely a benign cystadenoma. We have talked about cystadenoma, borderline and invasive tumors over the ovary, and certainly functional cystic mass could be present. We have talked on an endometrial biopsy; however, this may be perimenopausal or change in her bleeding pattern, but she does have a family history of small intestinal cancer in her father and in addition to her body habitus, she is at risk for endometrial hyperplasia. Therefore, this will be followed up. She wishes to proceed at least with laparoscopic unilateral salpingo-oophorectomy. She would like to save the contralateral ovary if a benign tumor is present. If an ovarian cancer was present, she understands both ovaries, tubes, and uterus should be removed. Should the biopsy of the uterus prove normal, she would like to pursue endometrial ablation at the same time. Risks of infection and bleeding were discussed with the patient in detail and a surgical date will be set and a biopsy will be followed up.

Electronically signed by John Andrews, MD. 1/1/20XX

**John Andrews, MD**

**Women's Cancer Center**

**1017 Rose Garden Ln.**

**Burley, ID 83768**

**DATE:** 01/01/20XX

**John, Thompson, MD:**

**RE:** Smith, Amanda

Dear Dr. Thompson,

I am writing to you regarding Amanda Smith, who as you know, is a 46-year-old sent by yourself for an adnexal mass. I had the pleasure of meeting her on 01/01/20XX. Please see my enclosed dictation. In summary, I have recommended the removal of the mass. It appears to represent a benign etiology and should that be the case, she would like to preserve her contralateral ovary and uterus. She has had likely perimenopausal bleeding but is at risk for endometrial neoplasm and an endometrial biopsy has been performed, the results of which are pending at this time. I will certainly keep you updated as to our findings and progress and very much appreciate the opportunity to become involved in your patient's care.

Warmest regards,

John Andrews, MD 1/1/20XX

# CASE 34

## *Transurethral*

**John Andrews, MD**

**Surgery Center**

**1017 Rose Garden Ln.**

**Burley, ID 83768**

**PATIENT:** Darrin Smith

**SEX:** Male

**AGE:** 65

**DATE OF SERVICE:** 01/01/20XX

**PREOPERATIVE DIAGNOSIS:** Transitional cell carcinoma of the bladder.

**POSTOPERATIVE DIAGNOSIS:** Transitional cell carcinoma of the bladder.

**PROCEDURE PERFORMED:** Cystourethroscopy, transurethral biopsies of the bladder and prostate urethra.

Anesthesiologist, LK, MD personally provided the general endotracheal anesthesia for the case while directing five CRNAs (PS IV)

LL, CRNA placed a non-tunneled central venous catheter in the left internal jugular vein at the beginning of the case

**Anesthesia start time:** 9:50 A.M. **Anesthesia end time:** 11:15 A.M.

The case, according to the anesthesiologist was complicated by utilization of controlled hypotension.

**SURGEON:** John Andrews, MD

**DESCRIPTION OF PROCEDURE:** The patient was taken to the operating room, placed on the operating table and given a general anesthetic. The patient was placed in the lithotomy position where the genitalia was prepped and draped in the usual sterile manner.

A #23 French cystoscope passed through the urethra under direct visualization revealing no abnormalities throughout the entire urethra until I reached the prostatic urethra. The fossa was patent and there was no evidence of partial resection of the prostate. On the right lateral lobe in the distal portion and was some area that looked almost edematous, but no tumor. There was an area along the bladder neck especially on the patient's right side that looked a little granular in appearance, but no obvious tumor. Within the bladder, there were some multiple areas of well-healed scars from previous tumors, but no indication of any recurrence in any of those regions. The left ureteral orifice was perfectly normal. The right ureteral orifice was a little flattened, but no tumors seen in either region. There was only one region on the left posterior wall of the bladder wall that had a tiny reddish area, but no tumors were seen throughout the bladder circumference. Using the biopsy forceps, pieces of the bladder mucosa were taken from the right posterior wall of the bladder and the left posterior wall of the bladder including the little reddish area previously mentioned. Those were sent in separate specimens and then biopsies were also taken from the bladder neck and prostatic urethra area in those regions previously described and those were submitted as a third specimen. The regions just mentioned were thoroughly cauterized with a Bugby electrode. There was no bleeding. The area was thoroughly irrigated with sterile water. Noted was some white flaky material floating around from the instrumentation and it appeared to be coming from the prostatic urethra as if old necrotic tissue was sloughing off. Once the bladder was thoroughly irrigated, all instruments were removed.

The patient was taken to the recovery room in good condition. There was no blood loss.

Electronically signed by John Andrews, MD. 1/1/20XX

**John Andrews, MD**

**Surgery Center**

**1017 Rose Garden Ln.**

**Burley, ID 83768**

**PATIENT:** Darrin Smith

**AGE:** 65

**DATE OF SERVICE:** 01/01/20XX

**HISTORY OF PRESENT ILLNESS:** This is a 65-year-old male who has been here a few times for bladder tumor. His history has not changed significantly in that he had his original tumors in 2010 and had multiple sites. They never did show invasion but did have some recurrences. He underwent ECG treatments which eventually failed, so went to the Valstar bladder instillation treatment. They seemed to work very well except just recently so it appeared that he may have an early tumor trying to come back again. I have had an e-mail with Dr. Kramer regarding his treatment. His recent cystoscopy did not show any definite tumors, but his urine cytology showed what appeared to be some malignant cells. He is brought in at this time for bladder biopsy. His renal function studies including BUN and creatinine have been slightly increasing lately, so I will later want an ultrasound of his kidneys to check for any hydronephrosis or other abnormalities.

**PAST MEDICAL HISTORY:** No significant change.

**MEDICATIONS:** Nexium.

**ALLERGIES:** PENICILLIN.

**SOCIAL HISTORY:** Never smoked and does have an occasional alcoholic beverage.

**REVIEW OF SYSTEMS:** No complaints except some upper respiratory allergies periodically.

**PHYSICAL EXAMINATION:**

**GENERAL:** Vital signs as listed in the chart. **HEENT:** Normal to inspection forage.

**CHEST:** Symmetrical.

**LUNGS:** Clear to auscultation.

**HEART:** No evidence of cardiomegaly, murmurs or rhythm irregularities.

**ABDOMEN:** Soft, no masses palpable.

**EXTERNAL GENITALIA:** Normal adult male.

**IMPRESSION:** Transitional cell carcinoma of the bladder.

Electronically signed by John Andrews, MD. 1/1/20XX

**Pathology Center**

**1017 Rose Garden Ln.**

**Burley, ID 83768**

**PATIENT:** Darrin Smith

**AGE:** 65

**DATE COLLECTED:** 01/01/20XX

**DATE RECEIVED:** 01/01/20XX

**DATE REPORTED:** 01/04/20XX

**CLINICAL INFORMATION:**

Bladder cancer.

**DIAGNOSIS:**

A. Right posterior bladder wall biopsy: Benign urinary bladder tissue.
B. Left posterior bladder wall, biopsy: Benign urinary bladder tissue.
C. Prostatic urethra, biopsy: Benign squamous mucosa.

**SPECIMENS:** Posterior wall bladder right side, posterior wall bladder left side, prostate urethra

**GROSS DESCRIPTION:** Specimen A is labeled with the patient's name and "right posterior wall bladder". Received in formalin is a single pink-tan, irregular rubbery tissue fragment measuring 0.2 x 0.1 by less than 0.1 cm. The remaining formalin is forwarded to cytology for cytospin preparation.

Specimen B is labeled with the patient's name and "left posterior bladder wall". Received in formalin is a single pink-tan, irregular rubbery tissue fragments measuring 0.2 x 0.1 by less than 0.1 cm. The remaining formalin is forwarded to cytology for cytospin preparation.

Specimen C is labeled with the patient's name and "prostate urethra x2". Received in formalin are 2-minute pale tan, irregular soft tissue fragments measuring 0.2 x 0.2 by less than 0.1 cm in aggregate. The specimen may not survive processing.

**MICROSCOPIC DESCRIPTION:** A-C complete microscopic examination is performed.

Electronically signed by John Kramer, MD. 1/1/20XX

# CASE 35

## *Integumentary system, muscles, and nerves*

**John Andrews, MD**

**Surgery Center**

**1017 Rose Garden Ln.**

**Burley, ID 83768**

**PATIENT:** Roger Smith

**SEX:** Male

**AGE:** 44

**DATE OF SERVICE:** 01/01/20XX

**PREOPERATIVE DIAGNOSES:** Painful mass of right thumb.

**POSTOPERATIVE DIAGNOSES:** Epidermal cyst with associate neuroma of an amputated stump of right thumb.

**PROCEDURE:** Exploration of right thumb with excision of cystic mass 2.2 cm with 0.5 cm margins, contouring of bone, revision of amputation stump, excision of bilateral neuromas, application of the soft dressing.

**SURGEON:** John Andrews, MD

**ANESTHESIOLOGIST:** John Kramer, MD personally provided the general endotracheal anesthesia for the case (PS II)

JK, MD placed a Swan-Ganz catheter for monitoring purposes at the beginning of the case. The anesthesiologist JK, MD also performed echocardiography, transesophageal, real-time with image documentation (2D), including probe placement, image acquisition, interpretation and report during the case.

**Anesthesia start time:** 9:37 A.M. **Anesthesia end time:** 12:15 P.M.

**ANESTHESIA:** General endotracheal anesthesia.

**INDICATION:** This 44-year-old right-hand dominant butcher had sustained a work-related injury in 2010 in which he sustained a partial amputation of the right thumb and also an injury to the right index finger. He underwent repair with revision amputation of the right thumb and repair of nerve and tendon of the right index finger. He had been doing well until last fall when the right thumb showed evidence of an irritative growth which became painful and irritative and also occasionally drained some purulent material. It was suspected that this represented some type of granuloma epidermal cyst possibly with associated neuroma since it was quite tender on the projected portion of the mass. He presents now for operative exploration with excision of the mass which could also be retained nail bed matrix and any associated neuroma.

**DESCRIPTION OF PROCEDURE:** The patient was prepped and draped in the usual fashion. Under satisfactory general anesthesia with a tourniquet in place, the right upper extremity was exsanguinated and the tourniquet was inflated to 250 mmHg. With the marking pen, an ellipse was drawn about the mass and also along the previous scar at the amputation stump. The mass was located on the radial aspect of the thumb. Then with a 15C blade, an incision was made. Dissection proceeded down through the skin and subcutaneous tissue and a pearly cystic wall was encountered, likely the cyst present. This was carefully dissected and 3.9 cm was removed and passed off for pathology. The flap that had been used to repair the thumb was taken down and there was evidence of some irritative nerve stump. This was then dissected out with fine Iris scissors, grasped and placed on stretch and the base was then resected to allow retraction into the soft tissue thumb pad. A rongeur was used to help further mold the bone. The ulnar side of the thumb was also explored and a small nerve stump was found and resected in a similar fashion to the radial side. The wound was irrigated. There did not appear to be any other foreign body or cystic elements present. The wound was then closed with interrupted horizontal mattress 5-0 black nylon suture in a 2.25 cm intermediate repair. Further modification of the skin was made in order to help contour the radial side of the thumb soft tissue which had been expanded by the cyst and then a 6-0 Prolene was used to further close the edges of the skin over the thumb tip. The tourniquet was released. A block consisting of 0.5% plain Marcaine was injected at the base of the thumb. The wound was cleaned and dressed in Xeroform, bacitracin, fluffs, tube gauze, and a 2-inch Ace wrap.

The patient was then extubated and taken to the recovery area in good condition.

Electronically signed by John Andrews, MD.

**John Andrews, MD**

**Surgery Center**

**1017 Rose Garden Ln.**

**Burley, ID 83768**

**PATIENT:** Roger Smith

**AGE:** 44

**Medicare-Payer**

**DATE OF SERVICE:** 01/01/20XX

**CHIEF COMPLAINT:** Mass on amputation stump, right thumb.

**HISTORY OF PRESENT ILLNESS:** A 44-year-old male butcher with a work-related injury, right hand with an injury to right thumb and index finger status post revision amputation right thumb, now with a mass on amputation stump, presents for excision.

**PAST SURGICAL HISTORY:** Surgery right hand, 20XX.

**ALLERGIES:** NKDA.

**PHYSICAL EXAMINATION: EXTREMITIES:** Surgery right hand. Mass on the right thumb.

**IMPRESSION:** Mass right thumb.

**PLAN:** Excise mass right thumb.

Electronically signed by John Andrews, MD. 1/1/20XXX

**Pathology Center**

**1017 Rose Garden Ln.**

**Burley, ID 83768**

**PATIENT:** Roger Smith

**AGE:** 44

**Collected:** 01/01/20XX

**Received:** 01/0/20XX

**Reported:** 01/01/20XX

**CLINICAL INFORMATION:**

Right thumb mass.

**DIAGNOSIS:**

FIBROADIPOSE TISSUE (RIGHT THUMB MASS): BENIGN SQUAMOUS EPITHELIAL INCLUSION CYST.

**SPECIMENS:** RIGHT THUMB MASS

**GROSS DESCRIPTION:**

Received labeled "right thumb mass" are pale pinkish tan pieces of soft and firm tissue that measure in the aggregate 2 x 1.5 x 0.4 cm. The entire specimen is submitted in one cassette.

**MICROSCOPIC DESCRIPTION:**

All stains and controls are adequate.

Electronically signed by John Kramer, MD 1/1/20XXX

# CASE 36

## Bones of the lower leg, ankle, and foot

**John Andrews, MD**

**Surgery Center**

**1017 Rose Garden Ln.**

**Burley, ID 83768**

**PATIENT:** Hannah Smith

**SEX:** Male

**AGE:** 37

**DATE OF SERVICE:** 01/01/20XX

This is a Commercial Payer

**OPERATIVE REPORT**

**PREOPERATIVE DIAGNOSIS:**

1. Right ankle distal fibula lateral malleolus fracture.
2. Right ankle syndesmotic ligament tear.

**POSTOPERATIVE DIAGNOSIS:**

1. Right ankle distal fibula and lateral malleolus fracture.
2. Right ankle syndesmotic ligament tear.
3. Stable right ankle posterior malleolus fracture.

**PROCEDURE PERFORMED:**

1. Open treatment internal fixation right fibula lateral malleolus fracture.
2. Open treatment with internal fixation right ankle syndesmosis.

**SURGEON:** John Andrews, MD 1/1/20XX

**ASSISTANT:** John Thompson, MD

**ANESTHESIOLOGIST:** John Kramer, MD personally provided the anesthesia for the case (PS III)

**ANESTHESIA:** General endotracheal

**Anesthesia start time:** 8:50 A.M. **Anesthesia end time:** 11:47 A.M.

**COMPLICATIONS:** Anesthesia was complicated by utilization of total body hypothermia

**ESTIMATED BLOOD LOSS:** 30 mL.

**TOURNIQUET TIME:** 54 minutes at 300 mmHg.

**SPECIMEN:** None.

**FINDINGS:** Displaced right ankle distal fibula Weber C fracture as well as a syndesmotic ligament tear

**ORTHOPEDIC IMPLANT:** Synthes one-third tubular locking plate, with 2 individual 3.5 mm shaft screws, two individual 3.5 mm cortex screws, four individual 3.5 mm locking screws and a 4.5 mm cortex screw.

**INDICATIONS:** This is a 37-year-old male who injured his right ankle at work (warehouse) 4 weeks ago. He was diagnosed with a right ankle distal fibula Weber C fracture as well as a syndesmotic ligament tear. The diagnosis, treatment options, risks, and benefits were discussed with the patient. Because of the unstable nature of the fracture, associated with the Weber C fracture and the syndesmotic ligament tear, it was recommended to proceed with open treatment with internal fixation of the fracture to allow for stabilization of the fracture as well as to assess and treat the syndesmotic ligament tear with a syndesmotic screw as indicated. The details of the procedure were discussed with the patient using lay terms to the best of my ability, including the risks and benefits and expected outcomes. The risks of the procedure include but are not limited to bleeding, infection, blood clot, pain, swelling, numbness, stiffness or arthritis of the ankle. The risks also include injury to blood vessels, nerves, ligaments, tendons, muscle, cartilage or bone of the ankle. The risks also include foot drop or deformity of the ankle, fracture nonunion or fracture malunion, hardware irritation requiring removal or the need for additional ankle surgery. The patient verbalized understanding of this and gave his written consent.

**DESCRIPTION OF PROCEDURE:** The patient was taken to the operative suite under the guidance of anesthesia and placed in the supine position on the operating table. After appropriate general anesthesia had been given, a tourniquet was placed high on the right thigh. The right lower extremity was sterilely prepped and draped in the usual sterile fashion. The right lower extremity was exsanguinated and the tourniquet was inflated to 300 mmHg.

C-arm fluoroscopy verified the patient's right ankle distal fibula and lateral malleolus Weber C fracture. A longitudinal incision was made over the lateral aspect of the right distal fibula, centered over the fracture site. Careful blunt and sharp dissection was carried through the subcutaneous tissues with electrocautery used as needed to help achieve hemostasis. The deep fascial tissue was excised and the dissection was extended down to the fracture site. The fracture was found to be comminuted with a large butterfly fragment. There was a large and long oblique fracture fragment. There was a large and long oblique fracture fragment that extended up the distal fibula shaft. The fracture was debrided and irrigated. The fracture was reduced and held reduced with a bone reduction clamp.

Initial stabilization was performed with the use of 2 individual 3.5 mm shaft screws, used as interfragmentary screws. These were placed in the standard technique of drilling both cortices over drilling the near cortex and placing the appropriate length 3.5 mm shaft screw. These achieved good initial fixation at the fracture.

Attention was then turned to the placement of a one-third tubular locking plate along the lateral aspect of the lateral malleolus fracture. Because of the long oblique nature of this fracture, a longer plate was necessary. Therefore a 10-hole one-third tubular locking plate was contoured against the lateral aspect of the distal fibula. This was initially stabilized with the placement of a 3.5 mm cortex screw proximal to the fracture. This was placed in the standard technique of drilling both cortices, measuring and placing the appropriate length 3.5 mm cortex screw with good fixation. Because this initial screw was at the site of the long posterior fracture fragment, I chose to proceed with 3 additional screws proximal to this. Therefore 3 individual 3.5 mm locking screws were placed in the three most proximal holes of the one-third tubular locking plate. These were placed in the standard technique of drilling both cortices, measuring and placing the appropriate length 3.5 mm locking screw. These all achieved good fixation and good stabilization.

Attention was then turned to the placement of screws distal to the fracture. Two individual 3.5 mm locking screws were placed in the standard technique of drilling both cortices, measuring and placing the appropriate length 3.5 mm locking screw.

The distal hole of the one-third tubular locking plate was left empty. Cotton stress was then performed and there was found to be widening of the right ankle syndesmosis with loss of the normal tibia/fibula overlap on the mortise view x-ray. Therefore the decision was made to perform internal fixation for the syndesmosis ligament tear.

With the right ankle dorsiflexed, a periarticular bone reduction clamp was used to reduce the syndesmosis. This was verified with C-arm fluoroscopy. A drill hole was then placed through the distal fibula and into the distal tibia, approximately 2.5 cm proximal to the ankle mortise and parallel to the joint. This was measured and a 4.5 mm cortex screw was placed in the distal hole of the one-third tubular locking plate and through all 4 cortices of the distal fibula and tibia, thereby getting a good fixation and reduction of the right ankle syndesmosis.

The clamp was removed. C-arm fluoroscopy verified in the AP, the mortise and the lateral views that the fracture had been reduced to a near anatomic position with good fixation provided. There was a good reduction of the right ankle syndesmosis as checked with stress test x-rays under C-arm fluoroscopy. There was positive tibia/fibula overlap on the mortise view x-ray.

It also should be noted that with the lateral view x-ray there was a visualization of a very small posterior malleolus fracture fragment. This did not extend into the articular surface and the fracture was nondisplaced.

The tourniquet was deflated. Bipolar electrocautery was used as needed to help achieve hemostasis. The wound was thoroughly irrigated using copious amounts of normal saline under pulsatile lavage.

The deep fascial tissues were approximated using 0 Vicryl suture. The subcutaneous tissues were approximated using 2-0 Vicryl. The skin edges were approximated using 3-0 nylon. A sterile dressing was applied to the patient's right ankle, followed by the placement of a very well-padded right ankle posterior splint with stirrups. All instrument, needle and sponge counts were correct. The patient tolerated the procedure well and was transported to the postanesthesia care unit under the guidance of anesthesia in stable and satisfactory condition.

Electronically signed by John Andrews, MD. 1/1/20XX

**John Andrews, MD**

**Surgery Center**

**1017 Rose Garden Ln.**

**Burley, ID 83768**

**PATIENT:** Hannah Smith

**SEX:** Male

**AGE:** 37

**DATE OF SERVICE:** 01/01/20XX

This is a Commercial Payer (Follow Medicare rules. External causes are required)

**CHIEF COMPLAINT:** Right ankle and foot pain.

**HISTORY OF PRESENT ILLNESS:** This is a 37-year-old male who injured his right ankle and foot on 12/06/20xx. He fell and sustained a twisting injury to his right ankle and foot. He had an immediate onset of pain. He was examined in a local emergency department and he was diagnosed with a fracture. He was placed into a fracture boot. He has been partial weight bearing on the right lower extremity in his fracture boot using crutches. He apparently has already been examined by a local orthopedic surgeon; however, he presents to the office today for further evaluation of his right ankle and foot. He has been taking Tylenol as needed for pain. He describes pain with weight bearing on the right lower extremity localized the lateral aspect of the right ankle as well as to the dorsal aspect of the right foot. He also has swelling over the right ankle and the right foot.

**PAST MEDICAL HISTORY:** No medical history reported.

**PAST SURGICAL HISTORY:** No surgical history reported.

**FAMILY MEDICAL HISTORY:** No family medical history reported.

**SOCIAL HISTORY:** No tobacco or alcohol use reported.

**ALLERGIES:** No known drug allergies.

**MEDICATIONS:** Hydrocodone. Tylenol. Calcium OTC.

**REVIEW OF SYSTEMS:**

**CONSTITUTIONAL:** No fever or fatigue reported.

**HEENT:** No abnormalities reported.

**GASTROINTESTINAL:** No abdominal pain or liver dysfunction reported.

**NEUROLOGIC:** No headache or dizziness reported.

**INTEGUMENT:** No rashes or sores reported.

**CARDIOVASCULAR:** No chest pain or angina reported.

**GENITOURINARY:** No kidney disease reported.

**RESPIRATORY:** No shortness of breath or wheezing reported.

**MUSCULOSKELETAL:** Right ankle and foot pain.

**PHYSICAL EXAMINATION:**

**VITAL SIGNS:** Height 6', weight 180 pounds.

**GENERAL:** Awake and alert. No acute distress.

**HEENT:** Within normal limits.

**INTEGUMENT:** Skin is intact.

**NEUROLOGIC:** Cranial nerves II-XII are grossly intact.

**NECK:** Trachea is midline.

**CARDIOVASCULAR:** Regular rhythm.

**CHEST:** Normal breath sounds.

**ABDOMEN:** Non-protuberant.

**MUSCULOSKELETAL:** There is mild increased warmth and erythema noted over the dorsal aspect of the right foot as well as over the lateral aspect of the right ankle. There is 2+ pitting edema over the dorsal aspect of the right foot and 1+ pitting edema over the lateral aspect of the right ankle. Positive tenderness over the right ankle distal fibula, proximal to the ankle mortise. No tenderness over the medial aspect of the right ankle. Stress testing of the right ankle reveals it to be ligamentous stable. Positive tenderness over the dorsal aspect of the right foot in a diffuse pattern, centered over the metatarsals. No other tenderness noted over any other aspect of the right foot or ankle. Positive ecchymosis noted over the hind foot of the right foot and ankle. The patient can actively dorsiflex the right ankle to 10 degrees with active ankle plantar flexion of 20 degrees. Distally neurovascularly intact.

**RADIOGRAPHS:** Three view x-rays of the right ankle were performed on 12/06/20xx outside of the office and these images are available for review. This reveals a fracture of the right ankle distal fibula, proximal to the ankle mortise. This is a long, oblique fracture. The fracture is displaced laterally approximately 2 mm. There appears to be an incidental finding of an accessory ossicle adjacent to the distal fibula, which is chronic and not acute. No additional fracture noted over the ankle. The ankle syndesmosis appears to be intact with no medial clear space widening on the mortise view x-ray. There is still a slight tibia/fibula overlap on the mortise view x-ray.

Three view x-rays of the right foot were performed today on 12/15/20xx outside of the office. These x-rays are also available for review. This reveals no obvious fracture, dislocation or tumor.

**ASSESSMENT:** Right ankle distal fibula Weber C fracture.

**PLAN:**

1. The diagnosis, treatment options, risks, and benefits were discussed with the patient through the use of a Spanish interpreter as needed. The patient's fracture pattern appears to be a stable fracture. He has a minimal displacement of the distal fibula with no medial ankle injury. He has no tenderness over the medial aspect of the ankle with no medial malleolar fracture. I discussed with him that the level of his distal fibular fracture can be concerning for a possible syndesmotic ligament injury; however, on the mortise view x-ray, there is no medial clear space widening and there is still slight tibia/fibula overlap on the mortise view x-ray. Stress testing of the right ankle upon examination produces no pain over the syndesmosis.
2. Treatment options were discussed with him. This includes both a surgical and a nonsurgical treatment option. A surgical treatment option would involve open reduction with internal fixation of the right distal fibula fracture. The details of the surgery were discussed with him. An additional course of treatment would involve splint immobilization until the swelling improves, followed by cast immobilization. Details of this treatment option were discussed with him.
3. After a long discussion with the patient, carefully answering his questions, the patient would like to initially proceed with the nonsurgical treatment regimen. Therefore, he was placed into a well-padded right short leg posterior splint with stirrups. He tolerated this well.
4. He should keep the right foot elevated to decrease swelling and pain. He should be nonweightbearing on the right lower extremity with his crutches. He does not feel that he needs a medication stronger than Tylenol. He may also take an anti-inflammatory medication as needed under the supervision of his primary care physician.
5. I recommend reevaluation in the office in 1 week to check his progress. If his fracture continues to be in a stable position and his swelling has decreased, we can consider changing him into a short leg cast. I discussed with him that if his fracture displaces then we may need to consider surgical intervention. The patient agrees with this course of treatment.

Thank you so much for the recent referral of your patient for evaluation. Please do not hesitate to call for any questions or concerns. Again, I very much appreciate your referrals.

Electronically signed by John Andrews, MD. 1/1/20xx

H&P reviewed and there are no changes.

Electronically signed by John Andrews, MD. 1/1/20XX

## CASE 37

# Nerves, muscles, tendons, fascia, and bursae

**John Andrews, MD**
**Surgery Center**
**1017 Rose Garden Ln.**
**Burley, ID 83768**

**PATIENT:** Nancy Smith

**SEX:** Female

**AGE:** 32

**DATE OF SERVICE:** 01/01/20XX

Private Insurance (Medicare rules for 65 years and older)

**OPERATIVE REPORT**

**PREOPERATIVE DIAGNOSIS:** Left wrist soft tissue mass, possible ganglion cyst.

**POSTOPERATIVE DIAGNOSIS:** Left wrist soft tissue mass, ganglion cyst.

**PROCEDURE PERFORMED:** Excision of left wrist soft tissue mass, ganglion cyst.

**SURGEON:** John Andrews, MD

**ASSISTANT:** None.

**CRNAs:** 2 CRNAs LU, CRNA, JN, CRNA provided the anesthesia for the case (PS II)

**ANESTHESIA:** Monitored anesthesia care service

**Anesthesia start time:** 3:35 P.M. **Anesthesia end time:** 5:17 P.M.

**COMPLICATIONS:** None.

**ESTIMATED BLOOD LOSS:** 15 mL.

**TOURNIQUET TIME:** 14 minutes at 250 mmHg.

**SPECIMEN:** Left wrist soft tissue mass, ganglion cyst.

**FINDINGS:** Specimen findings of left wrist soft tissue mass, ganglion cyst.

**INDICATIONS:** This is a 32-year-old female with a left wrist mass over the dorsal aspect of her left wrist that has been present for approximately two and one-half years. This has not improved over the past two and one-half years. This seems to be getting bigger and she has some pain around the mass when she is lifting things or if there is pressure applied over the dorsal aspect of her left wrist. The soft tissue mass appears to be consistent with a ganglion cyst. The diagnosis, treatment options, risks, and benefits were discussed with the patient. Because she continues to have the mass, despite a conservative course of treatment, the patient has chosen to proceed with excision of this left wrist soft tissue mass. This would provide for a specimen to be sent to pathology to determine the extent of the soft tissue mass, which appears to be a ganglion cyst. The details of the procedure were discussed with the patient using lay terms to the best of my ability, including the risks and benefits and expected outcomes. The risks of the procedure include, but are not limited to Bleeding, infection, blood clot, pain, swelling, numbness, stiffness or arthritis of the wrist. The risks also include injury to blood vessels, nerves, ligaments, tendons, muscle, cartilage or bone of the wrist. The risks also include wrist drop, nerves, ligaments, tendons, muscle, cartilage, or bone of the wrist. The risks also include hand or wrist surgery. The patient verbalized understanding of this and gave her informed written consent.

**DESCRIPTION OF PROCEDURE:** The patient was taken to the operative suite under the guidance of anesthesia and placed in the supine position on the operating table. After appropriate general anesthesia had been given, a tourniquet was placed high on the left upper arm. The left upper extremity was sterilely prepped and draped in the usual sterile fashion. The left upper extremity was exsanguinated and the tourniquet was inflated to 250 mmHg.

Intraoperative examination of the patient's left wrist revealed a soft tissue mass over the dorsal aspect of the left wrist, over the radiocarpal joint. This was approximately 1.5 cm in diameter. A longitudinal incision was made directly over the soft tissue mass, over the dorsal aspect of her left wrist. Careful blunt dissection was carried through the subcutaneous tissues, with electrocautery used as needed to help achieve hemostasis throughout the procedure. The borders of this soft tissue mass were able to be identified. The extensor tendons for the left wrist were carefully protected at all times throughout the surgical procedures.

Once all borders of the soft tissue mass had been identified, the soft tissue mass was able to be excised from the left wrist. This included an extension of this soft tissue mass down to the dorsal wrist joint capsule which included a small but wide stalk. This soft tissue mass had the appearance and consistency of ganglion cyst. This was able to be excised, along with the stalk as well as a small portion of the dorsal joint capsule. This was excised and sent to pathology for the appropriate analysis.

The wound was thoroughly irrigated using copious amounts of normal saline. Further inspection of the left wrist revealed no additional sign of a soft tissue mass.

The tourniquet was deflated. Electrocautery was used as needed to help achieve hemostasis. The wound was irrigated using copious amounts of normal saline. Once again, further inspection of the wound revealed no additional sign of a soft tissue mass.

Once the wound had been thoroughly irrigated, the subcutaneous tissues were approximated using 2-0 Vicryl. The skin edges were approximated using 3-0 nylon. The skin and subcutaneous tissues of the left wrist were injected using 0.5% Marcaine plain without epinephrine for a total of 6 mL. A sterile dressing was applied to the patient's left wrist and secured with an elastic bandage. All instrument, needle and sponge counts were correct. The patient tolerated the procedure well and was transported to the postanesthesia care unit under the guidance of anesthesia in stable and satisfactory condition.

Electronically signed by John Andrews, MD. 1/1/20XX

**John Andrews, MD**

**Surgery Center**

**1017 Rose Garden Ln.**

**Burley, ID 83768**

**PATIENT:** Nancy Smith

**SEX:** Female

**AGE:** 32

**DATE OF SERVICE:** 01/01/20XX

Private Insurance (Medicare rules for 65 years and older)

**HISTORY AND PHYSICAL**

**CHIEF COMPLAINT:** Left wrist mass.

**ALLERGIES:** NKDA.

**HISTORY OF PRESENT ILLNESS:** A 32-year-old female with a left wrist mass x 2-1/2 years with no improvement with conservative treatment.

**PAST MEDICAL HISTORY:** Unremarkable.

**PAST SURGICAL HISTORY:** Right wrist ganglion cyst.

**SOCIAL HISTORY:** No tobacco or alcohol.

**FAMILY HISTORY:** Father with MI; a mother with HTN.

**LABORATORY DATA:** Noted in the chart.

**MEDICATIONS:** None.

**PHYSICAL EXAMINATION:**

**VITAL SIGNS:** BP 111/74, T 98.4, P 67, Right 18, weight 130 pounds, height 5 feet 2 inches.

**CONSTITUTIONAL:** No angina, no wheezing, no abdominal pain, left wrist mass.

**HEENT:** Within normal limits.

**NECK:** Within normal limits.

**LUNGS:** Normal breath sounds.

**HEART:** Regular rate and rhythm.

**ABDOMEN:** Soft, nontender, nondistended.

**BREASTS:** Deferred.

**RECTAL:** Deferred.

**PELVIC:** Deferred.

**EXTREMITIES:** Left wrist dorsal mass.

**SKIN:** Within normal limits.

**NEUROLOGIC:** Distally NVI.

**VASCULAR:** Within normal limits.

**LYMPHATIC:** Within normal limits.

**PSYCHIATRIC:** Within normal limits.

**IMPRESSION:** Left wrist mass, possible ganglion cyst.

**PLAN:** Excision left wrist mass, possible ganglion cyst.

Electronically signed by John Andrews, MD. 1/1/20XX

**John Andrews, MD**

**Surgery Center**

**1017 Rose Garden Ln.**

**Burley, ID 83768**

**PATIENT:** Nancy Smith

**SEX:** Female

**AGE:** 32

**DATE OF SERVICE:** 01/01/20XX

**DATE COLLECTED:** 01/01/20XX

**DATE RECEIVED:** 01/01/20XX

**DATE REPORTED:** 01/02/20XX

**CLINICAL INFORMATION:** Neoplasm of bone, left ganglion cyst.

**DIAGNOSIS:** Soft tissue, left wrist: Ganglion cyst.

**SPECIMENS:** Left wrist ganglion cyst.

**GROSS DESCRIPTION:** Submitted in formalin and labeled "left ganglion cyst" is an irregular fragment of rubbery dull grayish-tan tissue and attached fat measuring 2.0 x 1.4 x 0.8 cm. The outer surface is smooth and dull. Sectioning reveals a decompressed cystic structure containing smooth inner cyst walls. Entirely submitted in a single cassette. ONE BLOCK.

**MICROSCOPIC DESCRIPTION:** All stains and controls are adequate.

Electronically signed by John Kramer, MD. 1/1/20XX

CASE 38

# Moderate (conscious) sedation

**John Andrews, MD**
**Surgery Center**
**1017 Rose Garden Ln.**
**Burley, ID 83768**

**PATIENT:** Nancy Smith

**SEX:** Female

**AGE:** 59

**DATE OF SERVICE:** 01/01/20XX

Private Insurance (Medicare rules for 65 years and older)

**PREOPERATIVE DIAGNOSIS:** Bunion deformity right foot (hallux valgus)

**POSTOPERATIVE DIAGNOSIS:** Bunion deformity right foot (hallux valgus)

**PROCEDURE PERFORMED:** Bunionectomy with osteotomy and internal fixation right foot.

**SURGEON:** John Andrews, MD

**ANESTHESIOLOGIST:** John Kramer, MD personally provided the moderate conscious sedation for the case (PS III)

**Anesthesia start time:** 8:30 A.M. **Anesthesia end time:** 12:25 P.M.

**ANESTHESIA:** IV moderate conscious sedation.

**Intraservice time:** 3 hours 55 minutes

**DESCRIPTION OF PROCEDURE:** The patient was brought to the operating room and placed in the supine position. IV sedation was maintained throughout the entire procedure by anesthesia. Local infiltration of 0.5% Marcaine plain was injected in a Mayo fashion right foot. The right foot was then prepped and draped in the usual manner. Sterile technique was maintained throughout the entire procedure. With the foot prepped and draped, the right extremity was exsanguinated using an Esmarch tourniquet. AN ankle tourniquet was then elevated to 250 mmHg.

A 5 cm dorsomedial skin incision was made medial and parallel to the extensor hallucis longus tendon. The incision was deepened using sharp and blunt dissection. All bleeders were identified, isolated and ligated as necessary. A longitudinal incision was made over the dorsomedial aspect of the first metatarsophalangeal joint of the right foot. Using sharp dissection, the capsule was freed from underlying bony attachments on his medial and dorsal aspects. Exposure of the first interspace was achieved by going superficial to the extensor hallucis longus tendon. Using sharp and blunt dissection, the first interspace was exposed. A vertical capsulotomy was performed through the lateral capsule to the first metatarsophalangeal joint. The lateral collateral ligament suspending the fibular sesamoid was released. The adductor tendon was then released from the lateral aspect of the fibular sesamoid and the base of the proximal phalanx. It was noted at this time that the hallux was easily moved into the desired corrected position. Examination of the first metatarsal head revealed significant degenerative changes on the medial 25% of the first metatarsal head. The wound was copiously irrigated with Vancomycin solution. Vancomycin was also administered by anesthesia an hour prior to the procedure. The medial condyle and the first metatarsal head were remodeled using the sagittal saw. A transverse cut through the superior half of the first metatarsal head was made and slanted slightly proximally and exited the lateral cortex. The connecting inferior cut was made parallel to the metatarsal shaft exiting proximally to the metatarsal head. The capital fragment was then freed and moved up laterally into the desired corrected position. Two 0.045 K-wires were used to fixate the first metatarsal head in a corrected position. The pins were bent and cut and laid down next to the dorsal shaft of the first metatarsal. The medial aspect of the first metatarsal head was remodeled using a sagittal saw and an egg-shaped burr. The wound was copiously irrigated through the procedure. It was noted that the desired correction had been achieved. A 3 mm medial segment of the capsule was removed from the first metatarsophalangeal joint medially. A simple interrupted suture was placed in the plantar aspect of this excised area holding the hallux in a desired corrected position. Deep closure was finished using 4-0 Vicryl in a simple interrupted fashion. Skin closure was achieved using 4-0 Prolene in a horizontal mattress like fashion. Pictures were taken that showed the desired correction. The foot was dressed using Iodoform gauze, 4x4s, Kling, and Coban.

The patient tolerated the above procedure satisfactorily with the desired surgical results appeared to be achieved.

Electronically signed by John Andrews, MD. 1/1/20XX

**John Andrews, MD**

**Surgery Center**

**1017 Rose Garden Ln.**

**Burley, ID 83768**

**PATIENT:** Nancy Smith

**SEX:** Female

**AGE:** 59

**DATE OF SERVICE:** 01/01/20XX

Private Insurance (Medicare rules for 65 years and older)

**HISTORY AND PHYSICAL**

**CHIEF COMPLAINT:** Pain, right foot.

**HISTORY OF PRESENT ILLNESS:** The patient is being admitted to the Surgical Center for a bunion correction on her right foot. She has a history of a bunion correction on her right foot corrected several years ago and now she wants to proceed with surgical correction of the bunion on her right foot. She states that her blood sugar is under good control.

**PAST MEDICAL HISTORY:** She has a history of diabetes which is under control. Random blood sugar will be done preoperatively.

**MEDICATIONS:** She is currently taking Crestor, Zetia, Glucophage, Janumet.

**ALLERGIES:** She has a history of allergies towards PENICILLIN.

**PHYSICAL EXAMINATION: EXTREMITIES:** Lower extremities reveal skin temperature, texture, turgor and elasticity to be within normal limits bilateral lower extremities. She has well-healed scars on her left foot with good surgical correction. Her dorsalis pedis and posterior tibial pulses are +2/4 bilaterally. There is no edema to bilateral lower extremities. Her epicritic sensations are intact. Her muscle mass is symmetrical. Examination of her right foot reveals an abducting right hallux with a medially prominent first metatarsal head right foot. The first MPH range of motion has deviated and corrected position is smooth and pain-free. The prominence over the first metatarsal head is increasing according to the patient and according to my latest exam.

**ASSESSMENT:** X-rays taken in the office confirm the diagnosis of a bunion deformity on her right foot.

**RECOMMENDATIONS:** The patient is to go to surgery tomorrow for correction of bunion deformity on her right foot. Preoperatively her blood sugar will be checked.

Electronically signed by John Andrews, MD. 1/1/20XX

CASE 39

# Intraperitoneal

**John Andrews, MD**

**Surgery Center**

**1017 Rose Garden Ln.**

**Burley, ID 83768**

**PATIENT:** Victoria Smith

**SEX:** Female

**AGE:** 33

**DATE OF SERVICE:** 01/01/20XX

Private Insurance (Medicare rules for 65 years and older)

**SURGEON:** John Andrews, MD

**PREOPERATIVE DIAGNOSES:** Pelvic pain.

**POSTOPERATIVE DIAGNOSES:** Adhesions

**PROCEDURE:** Laparoscopic lysis of adhesions.

Anesthesiologist FD, MD performed the anesthesia for the case while directing 1 CRNA (PS III)

Anesthesiologist FD, MD placed a non-tunneled central venous catheter into the left internal jugular vein

**Anesthesia start time:** 11:00 A.M. **Anesthesia end time:** 12:20 P.M.

**ANESTHESIA:** General endotracheal.

**ESTIMATED BLOOD LOSS:** Less than 25 mL.

**OPERATIVE PROCEDURE:** The patient was taken to the operating room, administered general endotracheal anesthesia. The patient was then repositioned into the dorsal lithotomy position in Allen stirrups. The patient was then prepped and draped in the usual sterile fashion. The open-sided graves speculum was placed into the vagina and the uterine manipulator was then placed. Gloves were then changed and attention was turned to the abdominal portion of the case. Using a #11 blade, an infra-umbilical incision was created. The needle was inserted x 1 without difficulty. Hanging drop technique was used to establish intra-abdominal placement. Once this was confirmed, a pneumoperitoneum was established. Once adequate pneumoperitoneum was established, the varus needle was removed and a 5 mm trocar was inserted. Examination of the abdomen was performed and a 5 mm suprapubic trocar was placed under direct visualization. Examination of the pelvis was performed and post-procedural adhesions were noted in the Pouch of Douglas and the ovarian fossa. The harmonic scalpel was used to take down the adhesions. The tubes and ovaries were freely moveable. Excellent hemostasis was noted and the trocars were removed and the incisions were closed with 4-0 Monocryl and Dermabond. The instruments were removed from the vagina. The patient has awakened from anesthesia and transferred to recovery in stable condition.

Electronically signed by John Andrews, MD. 1/1/20XX

**John Andrews, MD**

**Surgery Center**

**1017 Rose Garden Ln.**

**Burley, ID 83768**

**PATIENT:** Victoria Smith

**SEX:** Female

**AGE:** 33

**DATE OF SERVICE:** 01/01/20XX

Private Insurance (Medicare rules for 65 years and older)

**CHIEF COMPLAINT:** Increased pelvic pain.

**HISTORY OF PRESENT ILLNESS:** Patient with increased left sided pelvic pain over the past 6 months. Patient with increased dyspareunia. Patient with normal US. IUD placed.

**PHYSICAL EXAMINATION:**

**General:** Normal.

**HEENT:** Normal.

**IMPRESSION:** Increased pelvic pain.

**PLAN:** DX lap.

Electronically signed by John Andrews, MD. 1/1/20XX

CASE **40**

# *Veins of lower leg*

**John Andrews, MD**

**Surgery Center**

**1017 Rose Garden Ln.**

**Burley, ID 83768**

**OPERATIVE NOTE**

**PATIENT:** Maria Smith

**SEX:** Female

**AGE:** 57

Private Insurance (Medicare rules for 65 years and older)

**DATE OF SERVICE:** 01/10/20XX

**PREOPERATIVE DIAGNOSES:** Varicosities of the left leg secondary to reflux of the anterior saphenous vein.

**POSTOPERATIVE DIAGNOSES:** Varicosities of the left leg secondary to reflux of the anterior saphenous vein.

**PROCEDURE:** Ligation and division of the left anterior saphenous vein followed by stab phlebectomy of the lower leg veins, a total of 11 incisions employed.

**SURGEON:** John Andrews, MD

**ANESTHESIOLOGIST:** John Kramer, MD performed the general endotracheal anesthesia for the case while directing 5 CRNAs (PS III)

The surgeon placed a central venous catheter into the right internal jugular vein at the beginning of the case.

**CRNAs:** NN, CRNA, JM, CRNA, JM, CRNA, ML, CRNA, SD, CRNA

**ANESTHESIA:** General endotracheal. The anesthesia was complicated by utilization of total body hypothermia.

**Anesthesia start time:** 8:35 P.M. **Anesthesia end time:** 11:15 P.M.

**ESTIMATED BLOOD LOSS:** Negligible.

**DESCRIPTION OF PROCEDURE:** The patient was taken to the operative suite and following induction of general anesthesia, was sterilely prepped and draped in routine fashion. Marcaine 0.5% with epinephrine was injected along our proposed line of incision through around an old scar in the left groin. An incision was then made through the old scar. Small bleeding sites were managed with electrocautery. Dissection was carried through the subcutaneous tissue with electrocautery. At this point, we identified the anterior saphenous vein. It was pretty well contained in all of the scar tissue. This was dissected out with blunt and sharp dissection. The vein was then isolated. It was then ligated with 2-0 silk and then divided. An additional vein was then seen coming off of the right side which was isolated and ligated with 3-0 silk. The deep femoral vein was identified lying adjacent to the femoral artery. This was left undisturbed. At this point, the deep tissues were reapproximated with interrupted 3-0 Vicryl followed by closure of the skin with a running subcuticular 4-0 Rapide Vicryl.

Attention was then drawn to the lower leg which had previously been demarcated in the holding area with a surgical marking pen. Multiple 2 to 3 mm incisions were3 then made with a #11 scalpel blade and hook phlebectomy technique was used to remove the vein in a piecemeal fashion. It was quite thickened and fibrotic and somewhat friable as we removed it. This was carried down to just above the medial malleolus. Following completion of this, the leg was cleaned. Then 0.25-inch Steri-Strips applied after placing Mastisol on either side of the incision. The leg was then wrapped using four-inch Kling and 4x4's followed by a six-inch Ace from the ankle up to the upper mid-thigh. The patient was subsequently awakened from the anesthetic and transferred to the recovery room in apparent satisfactory condition.

**GROSS PATHOLOGY:** This is a very pleasant 56-year-old female who had undergone a left greater saphenous vein stripping and had developed painful recurrent varices primarily in the lower anterior shin area. Repeat ultrasound had revealed the previously treated greater saphenous vein was removed. However, she has reflux in an anterior saphenous vein coming right from the saphenofemoral junction. This was then ligated today as well as stab phlebectomy to the veins in the anterior lower leg. There was also varicosity removed from the medial popliteal area.

Electronically signed by John Andrews, MD. 1/1/20XX

**Pathology Center**

**1017 Rose Garden Ln.**

**Burley, ID 83768**

**PATHOLOGY REPORT**

**PATIENT:** Maria Smith

**SEX:** Female

**AGE:** 57

Private Insurance (Medicare rules for 65 years and older)

**DATE OF SERVICE:** 01/10/20XX

**Collected:** 01/10/20XX

**Received:** 01/10/20XX

**Reported:** 01/11/20XX

**CLINICAL INFORMATION:**

**VENOUS INSUFFICIENCY:** VARICOSE VEINS, LEG PAIN

SEGMENTS OF VEINS WITH ADJACENT FIBROUS TISSUE (LEFT LEG): CONSISTENT WITH TISSUE WITH TISSUE FROM VARICOSITIES.

**SPECIMENS:**

VARICOSE VEINS FROM LEFT LEG

**GROSS DESCRIPTION:**

Submitted in formalin and labeled "varicose veins from the left leg" are multiple cylinders of grayish-tan tissues compatible with venous varicosities and aggregating to 2.5 x 1.6 x 1.3 cm. Representative sections are submitted in cassette A.

**MICROSCOPIC DESCRIPTION:**

All stains and controls are adequate.

Electronically signed by John Kramer, MD 1/1/20XX

# CASE 41

## Nerves, muscles, tendons, fascia, and bursae

**John Andrews, MD**
**Stone Hospital**
**1017 Rose Garden Ln.**
**Burley, ID 83768**

**PATIENT:** Smith, Marcus

**AGE:** 69

**DATE OF SERVICE:** 01/01/20XX

Private Payer (Medicare rules for 65 or older)

**OPERATIVE REPORT**

**PREOPERATIVE DIAGNOSIS:** Right carpal tunnel syndrome.

**POSTOPERATIVE DIAGNOSIS:** Right carpal tunnel syndrome.

**PROCEDURE PERFORMED:** Right open carpal tunnel release.

**SURGEON:** John Andrews, MD

**ASSISTANT:** None.

**ANESTHESIOLOGIST:** John Thompson, MD personally performed the monitored anesthesia care service for the case (PS II)

**ANESTHESIA:** Right upper extremity Bier block with monitored anesthesia care service

**Anesthesia start time:** 9:25 A.M. **Anesthesia end time:** 10:32 A.M.

Anesthesiologist placed a radial arterial catheter in the right radial artery at the beginning of the case

**COMPLICATIONS:** None.

**ESTIMATED BLOOD LOSS:** 20 mL.

The surgical procedure was deep complex, complicated, and markedly invasive.

**TOURNIQUET TIME:** 25 minutes at 250 mmHg.

**SPECIMENS:** None.

**FINDINGS:** Right median nerve entrapment within the carpal tunnel, consistent with carpal tunnel syndrome.

**INDICATIONS:** This is a 69-year-old male who has had numbness and tingling in the fingers of the right hand for the past few years and his symptoms are increasing. He has had a physical examination and electrodiagnostic study findings that are consistent with the right carpal tunnel syndrome. Because he continues to have symptoms despite a conservative course of treatment, he presented to my office for evaluation. The diagnosis, treatment options, risks, and benefits were discussed with the patient. Because he has continued to have symptoms despite a conservative course of treatment, the patient has chosen to proceed with an open right carpal tunnel release. The details of the surgery were discussed with the patient using lay terms to the best of my ability, including the risks and benefits and expected outcomes. The risks of the surgery include but are not limited to bleeding, infection, blood clot, pain, swelling, numbness, the stiffness of the right hand or wrist. The risks also include injury to blood vessels, nerves, ligaments or tendons of the right hand or wrist. Risks also include deformity of the right hand or wrist, recurrence of the right hand or wrist symptoms, a continuation of the right hand or wrist symptoms, or the need for additional right hand or wrist surgery. The patient verbalized understanding of this and gave his informed written consent.

**DESCRIPTION OF PROCEDURE:** The patient was taken to the operative suite under the guidance of anesthesia and placed in the supine position on the operating table. A tourniquet was placed high on the right upper arm. The anesthesiologist then gave a right upper extremity Bier block for the right upper extremity and the tourniquet was inflated to 250 mmHg. The right upper extremity was sterilely prepped and draped in the usual sterile fashion.

Anatomical landmarks were identified over the palmar aspect of the right hand. A longitudinal incision was made over the palmar aspect of the right hand, just ulnar to the thenar crease of the right hand, extending proximally to the wrist flexion crease. Careful blunt dissection was carried through the subcutaneous tissues, with bipolar electrocautery used as needed to help achieve hemostasis.

The dissection was extended down to the palmar fascia, which was incised in a longitudinal fashion. This allowed for visualization of the transverse carpal ligament. The proximal edge of the carpal ligament was identified. The neurovascular structures were carefully protected at all times throughout the surgical procedure. The ulnar aspect of the transverse carpal ligament was then incised from a proximal to distal direction, thereby performing the carpal tunnel release.

Once the carpal tunnel release was complete, the median nerve was inspected. Entrapment was found to be adequately released. There was no sign of any injury or synovitis present. There was found to be a good and complete release of the carpal tunnel.

The tourniquet was deflated. Bipolar electrocautery was used as needed to help achieve hemostasis. The wound was thoroughly irrigated with copious amounts of normal saline. The subcutaneous tissues of the right hand were approximately using 2-0 Vicryl. The skin edges were approximately using 3-0 nylon. The skin and subcutaneous tissues of the right hand were injected using 0.5% Marcaine plain without epinephrine for a total of 8 mL. A sterile dressing was applied to the patient's right hand, followed by placement of a very well-padded right volar wrist splint. All instrument, needle and sponge counts were correct. The patient tolerated the procedure well and was transported to the postanesthesia care unit under the guidance of anesthesia in stable and satisfactory condition.

Electronically signed by John Andrews, MD.

**John Andrews, MD**

**Surgery Center**

**1017 Rose Garden Ln.**

**Burley, ID 83768**

**PATIENT:** Smith, Marcus

**DATE OF BIRTH:** 01/01/1948

**DATE OF SERVICE:** 01/01/20XX

**HISTORY AND PHYSICAL**

**CHIEF COMPLAINT:** Right-hand numbness and tingling.

**ALLERGIES:** CODEINE.

**HISTORY OF PRESENT ILLNESS:** A 68-year-old male with right-hand numbness and tingling for a few years with increasing symptoms, no improvement with conservative therapy.

**PAST MEDICAL HISTORY:** Thyroid, allergic rhinitis.

**PAST SURGICAL HISTORY:**

**FAMILY HISTORY:** Father DM, MI; mother CA, liver disease. Siblings history of osteoarthritis, DM, osteoporosis.

**LABORATORY DATA:** Noted on the chart.

**MEDICATIONS:** levothyroxine, Estradiol, Protonix, Fosamax, Aleve, fluticasone, Zyrtec, vitamin D, fish oil, MVI, glucosamine chondroitin.

**PHYSICAL EXAMINATION:**

**VITAL SIGNS:** BP 159/79, T 97.5, P 93, R 18, weight 160 pounds, height 5 feet 8 inches.

**GENERAL:** No angina, no wheezing, no abdominal pain, right-hand tingling.

**HEENT:** Within normal limits.

**NECK:** Within normal limits.

**LUNGS:** Normal breath sounds.

**ABDOMEN:** Soft, nondistended, nontender.

**BREASTS:** Deferred.

**RECTAL:** Deferred.

**PELVIC:** Deferred.

**EXTREMITIES:** Right-hand carpal tunnel, tinels, positive Phalen sign.

**NEUROLOGIC:** Paresthesias right hand.

**VASCULAR:** Within normal limits.

**LYMPHATIC:** Within normal limits.

**PSYCHIATRIC:** Within normal limits.

**DIAGNOSTIC DATA:** EMG/NCV positive right carpal tunnel syndrome.

**IMPRESSION:** Right carpal tunnel syndrome.

**PLAN:** Right carpal tunnel release.

Electronically signed by John Andrews, MD. 1/18/20XX

# CASE 42

## Nerves, muscles, tendons, and fascia

**John Andrews, MD**

**Surgery Center**

**1017 Rose Garden Ln.**

**Burley, ID 83768**

**PATIENT:** Kirk Smith

**SEX:** Male

**AGE:** 33

This is a Commercial Payer (Follow Medicare rules. External causes are NOT required)

**DATE OF SERVICE:** 01/01/20XX

**OPERATIVE REPORT**

**PREOPERATIVE DIAGNOSIS:** Hematoma of the right leg.

**POSTOPERATIVE DIAGNOSIS:** Hematoma of the right leg.

**PROCEDURE PERFORMED:** Excision of deep hematoma right leg.

**SURGEON:** John Andrews, MD

**ANESTHESIOLOGIST:** Pinnacle Anesthesia. Anesthesiologist RW, MD personally performed the anesthesia for the case (PS II)

**ANESTHESIA:** General endotracheal.

**Anesthesia start time:** 7:00 A.M. **Anesthesia end time:** 8:50 A.M.

The anesthesia was complicated by emergency bleeding.

**GROSS PATHOLOGY:** The patient had an approximately 4-5 cm x 3 cm x 2 cm hematoma on the right leg just below the knee joint on the medial aspect of the leg just over the proximal tibial plateau region.

**DESCRIPTION OF PROCEDURE:** The patient had boxes fall on him 5 days ago (hematoma, need surgery) was taken to the operating room, placed in supine position and given a general anesthetic. The right leg was prepped with Hibiclens and draped in the usual orthopedic fashion. The leg was elevated, exsanguinated with an Esmarch bandage and a tourniquet was inflated to 300 mmHg on the high thigh region. Total tourniquet time for the procedure was approximately 30 minutes.

We made a transverse incision directly over the hematoma. The subcutaneous tissue was dissected sharply and bleeding was controlled with electrocautery. We observed the large hematoma and mass of scar tissue. We incised the fascia over it and then bluntly and sharply dissected it free from its surrounding tissue and from the joint capsule. It was excised in one piece and sent to pathology for analysis. It was incorporated with marked amounts of scar tissue and frayed and thickened fascial tissue. No signs of infection were present. The wound was then irrigated with sterile saline solution. A small rent in the joint capsule was closed using 0 Vicryl suture. The fascia was closed using 0 Vicryl suture. The subcutaneous tissue was closed using 3-0 Vicryl suture and the skin was closed using a running subcuticular 4-0 Rapide suture. Steri-Strips were applied to the wound. The wound was infiltrated with 0.5% plain Marcaine for postoperative analgesia.

A sterile compression dressing was applied and the patient was taken to recovery in apparent satisfactory condition. The patient tolerated the procedure well. The patient had no intraoperative complications. Estimated blood loss was 250 cc. Sponge, instrument and needle counts were correct.

Electronically signed by John Andrews, MD. 1/1/20XX

**FIRST ENCOUNTER**************************************************************************

**John Andrews, MD**

**Surgery Center**

**1017 Rose Garden Ln.**

**Burley, ID 83768**

**PATIENT:** Kirk Smith

**SEX:** Male

**AGE:** 33

This is a Commercial Payer (Follow Medicare rules. External causes are NOT required)

**DATE OF SERVICE:** 01/01/20XX

**CHIEF COMPLAINT:** Right knee pain.

**ALLERGIES:** Iodine.

**HISTORY OF PRESENT ILLNESS:** Today while working as a stocker in a retail store he was loading boxes on a truck and a stack of boxes fell and hit him on the inside portion of the right knee.

**PAST MEDICAL HISTORY:** Noncontributory.

**PAST SURGICAL HISTORY:** Noncontributory.

**FAMILY HISTORY:** Noncontributory.

**SOCIAL HISTORY:** Negative for tobacco, positive for ETOH 2 times a week, negative drugs.

**MEDICATIONS:** None.

**PHYSICAL EXAMINATION:**

**VITAL SIGNS:** BP 108/68, T 97.8, P 72, Right 14, weight 290, height 6'5".

**GENERAL:** Normal.

**HEENT:** Normal.

**NECK:** Normal.

**LUNGS:** Normal.

**HEART:** Normal.

**ABDOMEN:** Normal.

**BREASTS:** Deferred.

**GENITOURINARY:** Deferred.

**PELVIC:** Deferred.

**EXTREMITIES:** Right knee hematoma

**SKIN:** Normal.

**NEUROLOGIC:** Normal.

**VASCULAR:** Normal.

**LYMPHATIC:** Normal.

**PSYCHIATRIC:** Normal.

**IMPRESSION:** Right knee hematoma.

**PLAN:** Excise hematoma right knee.

Electronically signed by John Andrews, MD. 1/1/20XX

CASE 43

# Male genitalia

**John Andrews, MD**

**Surgery Center**

**1017 Rose Garden Ln.**

**Burley, ID 83768**

**PATIENT:** John Smith

**SEX:** Male

**AGE:** 12

Private Insurance (Medicare rules for 65 years and older)

**DATE OF SERVICE:** 01/01/20XX

**PREOPERATIVE DIAGNOSIS:** Phimosis and balanoposthitis.

**POSTOPERATIVE DIAGNOSIS:** Phimosis and balanoposthitis.

**PROCEDURE PERFORMED:** Circumcision.

**SURGEON:** John Andrews, MD

Anesthesiologist HS, MD performed the general endotracheal anesthesia for the case while directing one CRNA (PS II)

**CRNA:** LJ, CRNA

**Anesthesia start time:** 10:15 A.M. **Anesthesia end time:** 11:02 A.M.

**DESCRIPTION OF PROCEDURE:** The patient was taken to the operating room, placed on the operating table and given general anesthetic. The patient was placed in the supine position where the genitalia was prepped and draped to expose only the penis. The foreskin would not retract due to the severe phimosis, so a circumferential incision was made in the foreskin at the level of the corona. This was carried into the subcutaneous tissues. A dorsal slit was then performed and the foreskin was able to be retracted. There was quite a bit of meconium left in there from birth and this was cleaned off with Betadine. A circumferential incision was then made in the mucosa proximal to the corona and the 2 incisions connected in the midline. The foreskin with its subcutaneous tissue was then excised sharply and bleeding was controlled with coagulation. The skin and mucosal edges were then reapproximated with interrupted 4-0 Vicryl sutures. There was only minimal oozing of blood from the skin edge which was controlled with a bandage. In the frenulum was one little small bleeder which was cauterized. With the Telfa dressing applied, there was no visible bleeding. This terminated the procedure.

The patient was taken to the recovery room in good condition. Estimated blood loss was less than 25 mL.

Electronically signed by John Andrews, MD. 1/1/20XX

**John Andrews, MD**

**Surgery Center**

**1017 Rose Garden Ln.**

**Burley, ID 83768**

**PATIENT:** John Smith

**SEX:** Male

**AGE:** 12

Private Insurance (Medicare rules for 65 years and older)

**DATE OF SERVICE:** 01/01/20XX

**HISTORY AND PHYSICAL**

**HISTORY OF PRESENT ILLNESS:** This is an 11-year-old male whom I first saw in 2011. He has been having a lot of rash episodes under the foreskin and has a fair amount of phimosis making it difficult to keep the area under the foreskin clean. He has had no other health problems. Circumcision was discussed with him and his father and they wanted this done as soon as we could get it scheduled.

**PAST MEDICAL HISTORY:** The patient has had no other past medical disorders except for some allergy problems. He has had no prior surgeries or significant illnesses.

**MEDICATIONS:** Only Claritin.

**ALLERGIES:** He is not allergic to any medication known.

**SOCIAL HISTORY:** Negative.

**FAMILY HISTORY:** Negative.

**REVIEW OF SYSTEMS:** No other complaints.

**PHYSICAL EXAMINATION:** VITAL SIGNS: As listed in the chart.

**HEENT:** Normal to inspection for his age.

**CHEST:** Symmetrical.

**LUNGS:** Clear to auscultation.

**HEART:** No evidence of cardiomegaly, murmurs or rhythm irregularities.

**ABDOMEN:** Soft, no masses palpable and no tenderness elicited.

**EXTREMITIES:** No edema or deformity.

**EXTERNAL GENITALIA:** Testes are descended and normal to palpation. Penis: He has the phimosis as described with a history of infections under the foreskin.

**IMPRESSION:** Phimosis and balanoposthitis.

**PLAN:** Circumcision.

Electronically signed by John Andrews, MD. 1/1/20XX

CASE 44

# Integumentary system

**John Andrews, MD**
**Surgery Center**
**1017 Rose Garden Ln.**
**Burley, ID 83768**

**PATIENT:** Michael Smith

**SEX:** Male

**AGE:** 57

Private Insurance (Medicare rules for 65 years and older)

**DATE OF SERVICE:** 01/01/20XX

**DISCHARGE SUMMARY**

**ADMISSION DIAGNOSIS:** Seroma/lumbar spine surgical infection status post lumbar laminectomy, history of MRSA.

**DISCHARGE DIAGNOSIS:** Seroma/lumbar spine surgical infection status post lumbar laminectomy, history of MRSA.

**PROCEDURE PERFORMED:** Irrigation and debridement of the lumbar wound with intraoperative cultures.

**SURGEON:** John Andrews, MD

**INDICATIONS:** The patient is a 57-year-old white male who had a decompression lumbar laminectomy by me earlier in the month and did well with it and was able to go home as an outpatient. He started having increasing drainage, redness and temperature elevation.

**HOSPITAL COURSE:** He has been seen at the hospital. He comes back in the office with increased serous drainage from the area and I recommended hospitalization which was complete. He had a Gram stain performed that showed no epithelial cells, no white blood cells and no organisms seen. Later the Gram stain came back and showed many WBCs and a few RBCs, no bacteria were seen. Because of the patient's history of MRSA, he was started empirically on Vancomycin gram every 12 hours. He was placed on p.o. suppressive therapy with Doxycycline 100 mg every 12 hours and Rifampin 300 mg p.o. every 12 hours. This is as per infectious disease specialist that consulted later in the day. The patient's dressings were changed and the drain removed the first postoperative day. The incision site appeared to be clean and appeared to be healing well and the patient states he is having no pain. The patient is set up for IV antibiotic therapy and p.o. antibiotic therapy as per infectious disease.

**DISCHARGE INSTRUCTIONS:** The patient is to be seen back in the office at my facility in the near future for dressing change, wound inspection and re-examination. Questions or problems prior to that, the patient knows to contact us right away. The patient had a PICC line placed while here and that will be maintained through infectious disease staff as well.

Electronically signed by John Andrews, MD. 1/1/20XX

**John Andrews, MD**

**Family Clinic**

**1017 Rose Garden Ln.**

**Burley, ID 83768**

**PATIENT:** Michael Smith

**SEX:** Male

**AGE:** 57

Private Insurance (Medicare rules for 65 years and older)

**PROGRESS NOTE**

01/0X/20XX at 7:00

VSS, afebrile. Appreciate IDs note. Gram stain many WBCs, no organisms. Asked for PICC line. Dressings changed. Drain removed, new sterile dressings applied all under sterile technique. Progress satisfactory to date. The patient is planned for discharge to the home later today.

Electronically signed by John Andrews, MD. 1/X/20XX

**John Andrews, MD**

**Surgery Center**

**1017 Rose Garden Ln.**

**Burley, ID 83768**

**PATIENT:** Michael Smith

**SEX:** Male

**AGE:** 57

Private Insurance (Medicare rules for 65 years and older)

**PROGRESS NOTE**

**DATE OF SERVICE:** 01/01/20XX at 8:45 p.m.

**ID CONSULTATION**

SUBJECTIVE: Patient was seen and examined. Full consultation to be dictated. A 57-year-old male with SIRS, L spine wound infection status post I&D status post lumbar laminectomy, ____ MRSA set 1 x3 IV vancomycin.

**PLAN:**

1. Given the patient's history of recurrent MRSA skin/soft tissue infection, will treat with 65 weeks of IV vancomycin then p.o. suppression with p.o. doxycycline 100 mg every 12 hours rifampin 300 mg p.o. every 12 hours x3-6 months.
2. PICC line.3. Outpatient IV antibiotics in the ID clinic.
4. Follow up on wound cultures.
5. _____ diagnosis based on clinical course and culture data.

Electronically signed by John Andrews, MD. 1/X/20XX

**John Andrews, MD**

**Surgery Center**

**1017 Rose Garden Ln.**

**Burley, ID 83768**

**PATIENT:** Michael Smith

**SEX:** Male

**AGE:** 57

Private Insurance (Medicare rules for 65 years and older)

**DATE OF SERVICE:** 01/02/20XX

**OPERATIVE REPORT**

**PREOPERATIVE DIAGNOSIS:**

1. Status post lumbar laminectomy L5 bilateral, recent surgery.
2. Seroma formation lumbar spine, rule out infection.

**POSTOPERATIVE DIAGNOSIS:**

1. Status post lumbar laminectomy L5 bilateral, recent surgery.
2. Seroma formation lumbar spine, rule out infection.

**PROCEDURE PERFORMED:** Irrigation and debridement of the lumbar spine with aerobic and anaerobic cultures and Gram stains STAT.

**SURGEON:** John Andrews, MD

**ASSISTANT:** John Thompson, MD

**ANESTHESIOLOGIST:** John Smith, MD

Anesthesiologist personally provided the general endotracheal anesthesia for the case (PS III). The surgeon placed the P.I.C.C. line, which was already in place before the beginning of the surgery.

**Anesthesia start time:** 11:35 A.M. **Anesthesia end time:** 2:20 P.M.

**ANESTHESIA:** General oral endotracheal.

The anesthesia was complicated by emergency bleeding.

**DRAINS:** One small Hemovac.

**ESTIMATED BLOOD LOSS:** 375 ccs.

**COMPLICATIONS:** None.

**INDICATIONS:** The patient is a 57-year-old white male well known to me as recently he has undergone lumbar spinal surgery with me at L5-S1 level 3 weeks ago. He had a Gill procedure resection of posterior elements at L5. This was done at Surgery Center. It was done as an outpatient and went home. He was seen back in the office with some slight drainage. He was on antibiotic therapy at that time of Keflex 500 mg one p.o. 4 times a day. The patient's history is complicated by a previous Methicillin-resistant Staph aureus or MRSA infection following a different procedure in the past. The patient had a PICC line and 6 weeks of IV antibiotic therapy until he cleared the infection or was told that he was "cured". The patient has a nasal swab done at the clinic that came back negative for MRSA despite these measures. The patient has presented to our office under the clinic for additional care because of this. The seroma has not stopped with conservative management and we recommended the above and informed consent obtained.

**DESCRIPTION OF PROCEDURE:** The patient was taken to the operating room, put on the operative stretcher and placed on the operating table in the supine position. He was given IV sedation, the patient was orally intubated by the anesthesiologist and general anesthesia administered. The patient was turned in the prone position on top of the padded Wilson frame component of the radiolucent Jackson table. A sterile dressing was applied and the lumbosacral area was sterilely scrubbed, prepped and draped with sterile linens. All bony prominences had been properly cushioned and weight relieved. There was some slight serous drainage from the superior and inferior end of the incision site. A #10 blade knife handle was used to make a longitudinal incision through the old surgical cicatrix and took aerobic and anaerobic cultures and Gram stain for immediate STAT processing and given to the circulating nurse for that to take place. Suction to the seroma was complete. There was no purulence. There was no odorous smell to the wound. There were no signs of violating the lumbosacral fascia. The sutures were removed so we were just to make sure we went down and looked down to the fascia and did not see any large seromas down in that area. It was copiously irrigated with 3000 mL of sterile saline using a Simpulse type power lavage unit, thoroughly evacuated of irrigate and suctioned dry. Soft tissues were debrided with 4x4s and curette and good bleeding tissues. The thoracolumbar fascia was closed in the midline using #1 Vicryl interrupted figure-of-eight stitch fashion and a running stitch of the same. The subcutaneous was closed with interrupted inverted sutures of 2-0 Vicryl and the skin was closed with 3-0 nylon in horizontal mattress sutures and covered with Xeroform and 4x4s. A small Hemovac drain was placed anterior to the thoracolumbar fascia prior to closure and exited proximally into the left. It was cut to the appropriate length and connected to the reservoir in standard fashion.

With the sterile dressings in place, the drapes were removed. The patient was discontinued from anesthesia, rolled back in the supine position on the recovery bed and transported to the recovery room in apparent satisfactory condition.

The patient tolerated the procedure well. There were no complications encountered intraoperatively. All sponge and needle counts were correct.

Electronically signed by John Andrews, MD. 1/1/20XX

**John Andrews, MD**

**Surgery Center**

**1017 Rose Garden Ln.**

**Burley, ID 83768**

**PATIENT:** Michael Smith

**SEX:** Male

**AGE:** 57

Private Insurance (Medicare rules for 65 years and older)

**DATE OF SERVICE:** 1/XX/20XX

**HISTORY AND PHYSICAL**

**CHIEF COMPLAINT:** Drainage, lumbar spine.

**HISTORY OF PRESENT ILLNESS:** Patient is status post microscopic endoscopic lumbar hemilaminectomy on left L4-5, discectomy L4-5 and L5-S1 and foraminotomy L4-5 and L5-S1 on the left that was performed 3 weeks ago. The patient states his low back pain is doing much better. He denies pain at this time. He states he was unable to walk or weight bear on his right leg on Sunday, 10 days later and had swelling and went to the ER. They did an ultrasound to rule out DVT and put him in a splint. He was able to weight bear on Tuesday.

Evidently, there was concern about possible DVT and the Doppler ultrasound was negative. No anticoagulation is needed. The LBP is much better since surgery.

**ALLERGIES:** SULFA DRUGS.

**MEDICATIONS:** Lisinopril HCTZ 20-25 mg tab, carvedilol 25 mg tablet, amlodipine, clonidine 0.1 mg/day patch, Diovan HCT 80-12.5 mg tablet, potassium CL 10 mEq tab SA

**PAST MEDICAL HISTORY:** Patient has a history of hypertension.

**PAST SURGICAL HISTORY:** Patient has a history of arthroscopy, right knee, arthroscopy, left knee, and left knee replacement.

**FAMILY HISTORY:** Father has a history of hypertension, cancer, coronary artery disease, and heart attack. Mother has a history of cancer. Sibling has a history of hypertension.

**SOCIAL HISTORY:** Patient is right-handed. The patient appears to be well nourished and in good health. The patient uses alcohol and caffeine. The patient does not use tobacco.

**REVIEW OF SYSTEMS: CONSTITUTIONAL:** Patient has a history of fatigue. **EYES:** Patient has a history of glasses or contacts.

**HEENT:** Normal auditory acuity, no nasal drainage or difficulty swallowing.

**CARDIOVASCULAR:** Patient has a history of high blood pressure.

**REPS:** No shortness of breath or cough.

**GASTROINTESTINAL:** No abdominal pain, heartburn, hepatitis or bleeding.

**GENITOURINARY:** No dysuria or hematuria.

**MUSCULOSKELETAL:** Patient has a history of joint pain and stiffness.**SKIN:** Patient has a history of sores, rashes, lumps, dryness, and itching.

**NEUROLOGIC:** No headache, dizziness or memory loss.

**PSYCHIATRIC:** No mood change, depression or nervousness.

**ENDOCRINE:** No thyroid enlargement, sweating or excessive thirst.

**HEMATOLYMPHATIC:** No bruising, swollen glands or anemia.

**IMMUNOLOGICAL:** Patient has a history of skin rashes and reactions to drugs.

**PHYSICAL EXAMINATION:**

**VITAL SIGNS:** BP 129/74, pulse 66, height 67 inches, weight 195 pounds.

**IMPRESSION:** Lumbosacral radiculopathy.

**PLAN:** Lumbar: Patient to discontinue Valium and will begin Percocet one every 4-6 hours as needed for pain. Patient and spouse will call our office on Tuesday to verify that he is feeling more alert after D/C of Valium. No work at this time. We will address RTW at the next appointment. Neurontin 300m g disp 30 sig 1 p.o. at bedtime. Celebrex 200 mg disp 30 sig 1 p.o. daily.

**MEDICATIONS PRESCRIBED:** Neurontin 300 mg 1 capsule p.o. t.i.d. Quantity 30. Refills 1.

Electronically signed by John Andrews, MD. 1/X/20Xx

# CASE 45

## *Eye*

**John Andrews, MD**
**Surgery Center**
**1017 Rose Garden Ln.**
**Burley, ID 83768**

**PATIENT:** Owen Smith

**SEX:** Male

**AGE:** 64

Private Insurance (Medicare rules for 65 years and older)

**DATE OF SERVICE:** 01/01/20XX

**PREOPERATIVE DIAGNOSIS:** Chronic angle-closure glaucoma, right eye, moderate.

**POSTOPERATIVE DIAGNOSIS:** Glaucoma angle closure glaucoma, right eye, moderate.

**PROCEDURE PERFORMED:** Express mini shunt implantation, right eye.

**SURGEON:** John Andrews, MD

**ASSISTANT:** None.

**ANESTHESIOLOGIST:** John Kramer, MD

Anesthesiologist personally performed the general endotracheal anesthesia for the case (PS III)

**Anesthesia start time:** 10:00 A.M. **Anesthesia end time:** 12:20 P.M.

**ANESTHESIA:** General endotracheal anesthesia

**INDICATIONS:** This patient has longstanding diabetes. He has developed neovascular glaucoma but responded. The neovascularization responded to treatment with medication. He was left with chronic angle closure glaucoma and remains at an elevated intraocular pressure level despite maximally tolerated medical therapy. He is at risk for vision loss and even blindness at this level of pressure. Therefore, Express mini shunt implantation is indicated.

**DESCRIPTION OF PROCEDURE:** The patient was given topical peribulbar anesthesia in the preoperative holding room. When adequate anesthesia was obtained, he was brought into the operating room and sterilely prepped and draped in the usual manner for intraocular surgery. A lid speculum was placed between the eyelids of the right eye. A 6-0 silk corneal fixation suture was used to rotate the eye downward. Subconjunctival injection of lidocaine with epinephrine was administered superiorly and an incision was made at the limbus with a blunt Wescott scissors. Dissection was carried out posteriorly and bipolar wet-field electrocautery was used as needed to keep the surgical area clean and dry. A small pledget soaked with Mitomycin C solution was placed underneath the Tenon's layer and allowed to expose for several minutes. It was then removed and the area was irrigated well with a balanced salt solution. A small debridement of the peripheral cornea was done at the area of the limbus and then the scleral flap was outlined with a #57 Beaver blade and dissected anteriorly into clear cornea. A paracentesis was made in the inferotemporal corneal quadrant. Provisc was placed in the anterior chamber. The flap was then lifted again. A 26 gauge needle was advanced through the peripheral cornea and into the anterior chamber underneath the flap and was visualized in the anterior chamber. A paracentesis was made in the inferotemporal corneal quadrant. Provisc was placed in the anterior chamber. A small injection of Provisc was administered as the needle was withdrawn. The Express device was brought into the field on its insertion device. It was inserted through the opening and appeared to be in good position. It was released from the inserter device uneventfully and was well situated in the scleral bed. The flap was brought back into its base and sewn closed with several 10-0 nylon sutures so as to limit flow. The conjunctiva was advanced anteriorly. A tenectomy was performed in the area of the flap and the conjunctiva was sewn at the limbus with several horizontal mattress style 8-0 nylon sutures. Two small button holes were identified during the closure process and these were each closed separately with a 10-0 nylon suture in a pursestring fashion. The wound appeared to be water tight at the completion of the closure. The residual Provisc was irrigated from the eye through the paracentesis site with balanced salt solution and the eye was left at a relatively normal pressure level by palpation, subconjunctival injections of Gentamicin and Decadron were administered inferiorly. The corneal fixation sutures were removed. The lid speculum was removed. A TobraDex ointment was instilled in the eye. The lids were closed and a light patch and shield were placed over the eye.

The patient tolerated the procedure well and left the operating room in good condition. There were no complications.

Electronically signed by John Andrews, MD. 1/1/20XX

**John Andrews, MD**

**Surgery Center**

**1017 Rose Garden Ln.**

**Burley, ID 83768**

**PATIENT:** Owen Smith

**SEX:** Male

**AGE:** 64

Private Insurance (Medicare rules for 65 years and older)

**DATE OF SERVICE:** 01/01/20XX

**CHIEF COMPLAINT:** Elevated intraocular pressure.

**HISTORY OF PRESENT ILLNESS:** At the risk of vision loss and even blindness.

**PAST MEDICAL HISTORY:** None.

**MEDICATIONS:** See medication reconciliation record.

**REVIEW OF SYSTEMS:**

**GENERAL:** Normal.

**HEART:** Normal.

**LUNGS:** Normal.

**EXTREMITIES:** Normal.

**GENITOURINARY/RECTAL:** Deferred

**PHYSICAL EXAMINATION:**

**VITAL SIGNS:** See chart.

**HEENT:** Normal.

**NECK:** Normal.

**NEUROLOGIC:** Normal.

**SKIN:** Normal.

**BREASTS:** Normal.

**ABDOMEN:** Normal.

**VASCULAR:** Normal.

**LYMPHATIC:** Normal.

**PSYCHIATRIC:** Normal.

**IMPRESSION:** Unremarkable. HIN (well controlled), DM (well controlled).

**PLAN:** Patient is cleared for glaucoma surgery.

Electronically signed by John Andrews, MD. 1/1/20XX

# CASE 46

## *Nerves, muscles, tendons, fascia, and bursae*

**John Andrews, MD**
**Surgery Center**
**1017 Rose Garden Ln.**
**Burley, ID 83768**

**PATIENT:** Jamie Smith

**SEX:** Female

**AGE:** 60

Private Insurance (Medicare rules for 65 years and older)

**DATE OF SERVICE:** 01/01/20XX

**PREOPERATIVE DIAGNOSIS:** Lymphadenopathy.

**POSTOPERATIVE DIAGNOSIS:** Lymphadenopathy, consistent with lymphoma.

**PROCEDURE PERFORMED:** Excisional biopsy left groin (femoral) lymph node.

**SURGEON:** John Andrews, MD

**ASSISTANT:** John Thompson, MD

**ANESTHESIOLOGIST:** John Kramer, MD personally performed the anesthesia for the case while directing 1 CRNA (PS III)

The CRNA placed a catheter in the right radial artery at the beginning of the case.

**CRNA:** LL, CRNA

**Anesthesia start time:** 7:00 A.M. **Anesthesia end time:** 8:25 A.M.

**ANESTHESIA:** General endotracheal.

**ESTIMATED BLOOD LOSS:** Minimal.

**OUTCOME:** She had an enlarged lymph node that was about 3.5 to 4 cm which was consistent with lymphoma by frozen section. A final diagnosis is pending permanent section.

**COMPLICATIONS:** None.

**SPECIMENS:** Lymph node from the left groin.

**INDICATIONS:** This is a 60-year-old female referred to me for a left groin lymph node that was enlarged. She has some other lymphadenopathy as well. She underwent a CT scan of the abdomen and pelvis with contrast; however, she had bilateral groin lymph nodes with a questionable mass on her bladder, but no retroperitoneal lymphadenopathy which would be more suggestive of lymphoma. Therefore, she was referred to Dr. Johnson of urology to evaluate her bladder. He did not see anything by cystoscopy. I recommended the excisional biopsy for definitive tissue diagnosis. The risks, benefits, and alternatives of surgery were thoroughly discussed with the patient in the office and informed consent was then obtained in the preoperative holding area.

**DESCRIPTION OF PROCEDURE:** After informed consent was obtained, the patient was identified in the preoperative holding area and the operative site was marked. She was taken to the operating room and placed in the supine position. General anesthesia was induced. The left groin was prepped and draped in the usual sterile fashion. A timeout was called confirming the procedure. Infiltration of local anesthetic was then performed in the skin and subcutaneous tissues and then a longitudinal incision was made directly over the palpable node, through the subcutaneous tissue.

Cautery was used to maintain hemostasis down to the subcutaneous tissue with the enlarged lymph node. This was carefully dissected out with both blunt dissections as well as between 3-0 silk ties. It was submitted for frozen section. The wound was irrigated with sterile saline. All bleeding points were cauterized. The wound was further infiltrated with local anesthetic, and then once hemostasis was achieved was closed with 3-0 Vicryl deep subcutaneous, 3-0 Vicryl superficial subcutaneous sutures and then a running 4-0 Monocryl subcuticular stitch. Derma bond was then applied x2 layers and then a sterile dressing over that.

The patient tolerated the procedure well, no complications. All lap, sponge and needle counts were correct at the end. She was awakened in the operating room and extubated and transferred to the recovery room in good condition. Final diagnosis pending permanent section, but by frozen section is consistent with lymphoma.

Electronically signed by John Andrews, MD. 1/1/20XX

**North Clinic**

**1017 Rose Garden Ln.**

**Burley, ID 83768**

**PATIENT:** Jamie Smith

**SEX:** Female

**AGE:** 60

Private Insurance (Medicare rules for 65 years and older)

**DATE OF SERVICE:** 12/15/20XX

**CONSULTATION**

**CONSULTING PHYSICIAN:** John Thompson, MD

**REQUESTING PHYSICIAN:** John Andrews, MD

**CHIEF COMPLAINT:** The patient is a white female. She was referred to us for consultation. She presents with lymphadenopathy.

**HISTORY OF PRESENT ILLNESS:** Complaint of lymphadenopathy. It began 2 weeks ago. It is of mild intensity. This is the first episode. Associated symptoms include 70-pound weight loss. She says the mass in her left leg does not hurt nor is it growing. She works at the school taking care of infants. She is a newly diagnosed diabetic. No family history of lymphoma. She does not have cats.

**REVIEW OF SYSTEMS: CONSTITUTIONAL:** Positive for unintentional weight loss. Negative for chills, fatigue, fever, night sweats, victimization by domestic violence or unintentional weight gain.

**EYES:** Negative for blurred vision, eye drainage, eye pain, use of glasses or contacts and photophobia.

**ENT:** Negative for ear pain, diminished hearing, tinnitus, frequent epistaxis, nasal congestion, nonhealing nasal ulcer, frequent rhinorrhea, bleeding gums, periodontal disease, use of dentures, hoarseness, oral sores/ulcers, sore throat, sore tongue, thrush and tooth pain.

**CARDIOVASCULAR:** Negative for chest pain, claudication, dizziness, orthopnea, palpitations, paroxysmal nocturnal dyspnea, pedal edema, tachycardia, and varicosities.

**RESPIRATORY:** Negative for recent cough, chronic cough, dyspnea, exposure to tuberculosis, hemoptysis, pleuritic chest pain, and frequent wheezing.

**GASTROINTESTINAL:** Negative for abdominal pain, acid reflux symptoms, anorexia, abdominal bloating, dysphagia, clay-colored stools, constipation, diarrhea, heartburn, hematemesis, hematochezia, hemorrhoids, melena, nausea, vomiting, odynophagia, and change in stool caliber.

**GENITOURINARY:** Negative for dysmenorrhea, dyspareunia, dysuria, lesions on external genitalia, hematuria, high risk sexual behavior, frequent UTIs, history of recurrent bacterial vaginosis, irregular menstrual cycle, menorrhagia, nocturia, polyuria, post-coital vaginal bleeding, post-menopausal vaginal bleeding, history of rape, history of sexual abuse, urinary incontinence, vaginal discharge and vaginal itching.

**MUSCULOSKELETAL:** Negative for arthralgias, back pain, joint stiffness, limb pain, and myalgias.

**INTEGUMENTARY/BREASTS:** Negative for acne, atypical moles, extremely dry skin, fungal nail infection, jaundice, pruritus, rash, wart(s), breast mass, skin changes of the breast, breast tenderness, nipple discharge and performance of self-breast exams.

**NEUROLOGIC:** Negative for ataxia, dizziness, fainting, headaches, memory loss, paresthesias, seizures, tremor, vertigo, and weakness.

**HEMATOLOGIC/LYMPHATIC:** Negative for easy bruising, excessive bleeding, history of blood transfusion and lymphadenopathy.

**ENDOCRINE:** Negative for increasing size of hands and feet, hair loss, temperature intolerances, hirsutism, hot flashes, increased skin pigmentation, infertility, polydipsia, polyphagia, development of striae and excessive sweating.

**ALLERGIC/IMMUNOLOGIC:** Negative for seasonal allergies, perennial allergies, frequent URI type illnesses, risk factors for HIV and urticaria.

**PSYCHIATRIC:** Negative for anxiety, crying spells, depression, feelings of stress, anhedonia, mood swings, personality change, premenstrual tension syndrome, difficulty concentrating, recreational drug use, sadness, sleep disturbance, and suicidal thoughts.

**PAST MEDICAL HISTORY:** Type 2 diabetes.

**GYNECOLOGIC HISTORY:** C-section x2 1980 and 1982, jaw surgery 1995, hemorrhoid surgery.

**FAMILY HISTORY:**

**Father:** Type 2 diabetes.

**Mother:** Healthy.

**Sister:** Medical history unknown.

**Paternal grandfather:** Medical history unknown.

**Paternal grandmother:** Medical history unknown.

**Maternal grandfather:** Medical history unknown.

**SOCIAL HISTORY:** Occupation: Teacher. She has never smoked, non-drinker. No substance abuse history.

**CURRENT PROBLEM:** Lymphadenopathy.

**ALLERGIES:** TRAMADOL; itching (adverse reaction).

**MEDICATIONS:** Metformin HCL, calcium.

**PHYSICAL EXAMINATION:**

**VITAL SIGNS:** height 5 feet 4 inches, weight 199 lbs, BMI 20.4, temperature 98.7, BP 116/60 mmHg (left arm, sitting), pulse 74 BPM (sitting).

**GENERAL:** Well developed and nourished; appropriately groomed, in no apparent distress.

**EYES:** Normal.

**ENT:** Normal.**NECK:** Supple, a full range of motion; no thyromegaly, no carotid bruits.

**RESPIRATORY:** Lungs clear to auscultation and percussion; symmetric expansion; no dyspnea.

**CARDIOVASCULAR:** Regular rate and rhythm. Normal S1, S2; no murmur, rub or gallop; normal PMI; 2+ carotid, radial, femoral, and pedal pulses; no aortic or femoral bruits.

**GASTROINTESTINAL:** Nontender, nondistended, no hepatosplenomegaly or masses; no bruits.

**LYMPHATIC:** Multiple left anterior cervical nodes (1-2 cm in size, firm, nontender, fixed); multiple right anterior cervical nodes (1-2 cm in size, firm, fixed); no supraclavicular nodes; left axillary node (1 cm in size, firm, mobile); right axillary node (1.5 cm in size, firm, mobile); right inguinal node (2.5 cm in size, firm fixed); multiple left inguinal nodes (1.5-3 cm in size, firm, fixed); exam witnessed by RN.

**BREAST/INTEGUMENT:** Skin: No sig rashes or lesions; no suspicious moles.

**MUSCULOSKELETAL:** Normal range of motion; strength and tone.

**NEUROLOGIC:** Cranial nerves, motor, and sensory function, reflexes, gait, and coordination are all intact.

**PSYCHIATRIC:** Appropriate affect and demeanor; normal speech pattern; grossly normal memory.

**ASSESSMENT:** Lymphadenopathy.

**ORDERS:** Computed tomography, abdomen, and pelvis; with contrast materials.

**PLAN:** I recommend an excisional biopsy of the left inguinal/femoral node with a frozen section for definitive tissue diagnosis. Risks, benefits, and alternatives to surgery were discussed. She understands and wishes to schedule. I recommend a CT scan first to image the extent of lymphadenopathy. I did inform the patient that I am suspicious of lymphoma.

**RADIOLOGY:** I have ordered CT abdomen/pelvis with contrast to be done.

**DIAGNOSIS:** Malignant lymphoma.

**COMMENTS:** Morphologically, the lymph node is totally effaced by a follicular lymphoid process comprised of small lymphocytes showing angulated and cleaved nuclei. This would appear to correlate with the flow-cytometry studies, which were verbally provided and will follow in a separate report. The case will be sent to Oncology Services for further immunophenotypic and morphological work-up. When these studies become available and addendum will follow.

Electronically signed by John Thompson, MD. 12/15/20XX

**Pathology Center**

**1017 Rose Garden Ln.**

**Burley, ID 83768**

**PATIENT:** Jamie Smith

**SEX:** Female

**AGE:** 60

Private Insurance (Medicare rules for 65 years and older)

**DATE COLLECTED:** 01/01/20XX

**DATE RECEIVED:** 01/01/20XX

**DATE REPORTED:** 01/01/20XX

**DIAGNOSIS:**

Left groin lymph node: Malignant lymphoma (see comment).

**COMMENTS:**

Morphologically, the lymph node is totally effaced by a follicular lymphoid process comprised of small lymphocytes showing angulated and cleaved nuclei. This would appear to correlate with the flow-cytometry studies, which were verbally provided and will follow in a separate report. The case will be sent to Oncology Services. For further immunophenotypic and morphological work-up. When these studies become available, and addendum will follow.

**SPECIMEN DATA:**

**SPECIMENS:** Left groin lymph node.

**FROZEN SECTION:** Consistent with lymphoma.

Submitted fresh and labeled "left groin lymph node" is a rubbery oval light grayish-tan fragment of tissue measuring 3.6 x 2.2 x 2.5 cm. The outer surface is smooth, glistening and grayish-tan. Sectioning reveals soft glistening light grayish-tan tissue with the overall appearance of fish-flesh. There are no areas of nodularity, discoloration or hemorrhage. A portion is submitted for frozen section analysis and in cassette FS. A generous portion is submitted for flow-cytometry analysis. Representative sections are submitted in 3 cassettes labeled A-C.

**THREE BLOCKS**

**DIAGNOSIS:**

B. Lymph node, left inguinal, excisional biopsy. Follicular lymphoma, follicular and diffuse pattern, low grade (grade 1-2 of 3).

**COMMENTS:** The inguinal lymph node biopsy shows the morphologic, immunohistochemical and flow cytometric features of follicular lymphoma. The lymphoma is low grade (grade 1-2), is composed of both follicular and diffuse components and shows the Ki-67 proliferation index of approximately 25%. There is no evidence of a higher grade process on this biopsy. If you have questions please call me.

**SPECIMEN DATA:**

Microscopic description:

B. Received are 4 H&E sections labeled FS, A, B, and C. All 4 sections show similar findings. The biopsy shows lymph node with a thin fibrous capsule showing infiltration into and beyond by lymphocytic infiltrate with similar features to those seen in the lymph node parenchyma. The lymph node parenchyma shows a vaguely nodular and diffuse infiltrate of predominantly small/medium-sized cells with mostly condensed chromatin and irregular nuclear contours. There are rare scattered centroblasts, but no significant numbers of histiocytes or dendritic cells are noted throughout most of the diffuse areas. Increased numbers of scattered mitoses are seen. Most of the vaguely nodular areas show the appearance of germinal centers with mostly similar small/medium cells are those described in the diffuse areas and without significant increase numbers of centroblasts.

An immunohistochemical panel was performed on block A and CD3, CD20, CD21, and Ki-67 are repeated on blocks FS, B, and C. A block A, CD3 and CD5 highlight scattered small T lymphocytes throughout the infiltrate. CD20 and PAX5 highlight the predominance of infiltrating cells and show coexpression with CD10, BCL6, and BCL2; these cells are predominantly negative with large regions showing few to none comprising approximately half of the total infiltrate. The Ki-67 proliferation index is relatively uniform throughout and is approximately 25%. The immunostains on blocks FS, B and C show similar findings to those describe3d above for block A, including scattered CD3(+) small T lymphocytes, a predominance of CD20(+) cells, CD21(+) meshworks scattered throughout the infiltrate with large areas lacking, and a uniform and similar Ki-67 proliferation index.

**INTERPRETATION:**

CD10 (+) B-Lineage Non-Hodgkin lymphoma

**COMMENT:** Flow cytometric analysis reveals a CD10 (+) B-lineage non-Hodgkin lymphoma of small to medium cell size. The differential diagnosis includes follicular lymphoma and diffuse large B-cell lymphoma. A conventional karyotype is in progress and will be reported separately upon completion.

If you have questions please call.

**MORPHOLOGY:** The cytospin, smear and touch prep preparations show a monotonous population of small to medium-sized lymphocytes, some of which show cleaved and irregular nuclei.

FLOW CYTOMETRIC FINDINGS:Abnormal cells: 76% small-medium (forward light scattered properties) B-cells characterized as positive are CD10, CD19, CD20, CD36, FM-7, and kappa; negative for CD5, CD23 and lambda.

**OTHER CELLS:**

1% polytypic predominantly small (forward light scatter properties) B-cells (CD19+, CD20+) kappa/lambda ratio= 1.5:1.

20% small T cells (CD3) with non-aberrant expression of pan T-cell antigens CD5 and CD7; CD4/CD8 ratio= 8.8:1.

<1% NK cells (CD3+, CD7+, CD56 variable+)

<1% plasma cells (CD38+).

Debris/CD45 cells compromise the majority of the remaining events.

SPECIMEN VIABILITY 99%.

**GENETIC ANALYSIS**

**SPECIMEN TYPE:** Lymph node

**CLINICAL HISTORY:** Lymphadenopathy, probable lymphoma by frozen section.

**INTERPRETATION:**

Abnormal cytogenetic result.

Six out of 13 metaphases showed a translocation between chromosomes 14 and 18. The majority of the abnormal cells exhibited additional numerical and structural abnormalities indicating clonal evolution and genetic instability.

The t (14; 18) has been associated with follicular lymphoma and with diffuse large cell lymphoma. The clonal evolution and genetic instability point to a high-grade malignancy.

Other clinical and laboratory evaluations may further define the condition of this patient.

**COMMENT:** Please expect the results of any other concurrent study in a separate report.

Electronically signed by John Kramer, MD. 1/1/20XX

**Radiology Center**

**1017 Rose Garden Ln.**

**Burley, ID 83768**

**PATIENT:** Jamie Smith

**SEX:** Female

**AGE:** 60

Private Insurance (Medicare rules for 65 years and older)

**DATE OF SERVICE:** 01/01/20XX

**PHYSICIAN:** John Andrews, MD

**EXAM:** X-ray chest PA and lateral.

**REASON:** Pre-op

**FINAL REPORT:**

Two views of the chest are submitted. No prior examination for comparison.

Normal heart size. Prominent interstitial markings probably reflect a degree of fibrosis. An acute pulmonary process is not seen. Moderate dorsal kyphosis.

**CONCLUSIONS:**

1. No acute process is seen in the chest. Prominent interstitial markings probably reflect a degree of fibrosis.

Electronically signed by John Andrews, MD. 1/1/20XX

# CASE 47

# *Hernia repairs*

**John Andrews, MD**

**Surgery Center**

**1017 Rose Garden Ln.**

**Burley, ID 83768**

**PATIENT:** Chad Smith

**SEX:** Male

**AGE:** 40

Private Insurance (Medicare rules for 65 years and older)

**DATE OF SERVICE:** 01/01/20XX

**PREOPERATIVE DIAGNOSES:** Incisional hernia at the epigastric trocar site from the previous cholecystectomy.

**POSTOPERATIVE DIAGNOSES:** Incisional hernia at the epigastric trocar site from the previous cholecystectomy with the defect measuring approximately 2-2.4 cm in diameter containing preperitoneal fat.

**PROCEDURE:** Incisional herniorrhaphy.

**SURGEON:** John Andrews, MD

**ASSISTANT:** John Thompson, MD

**ANESTHESIOLOGIST:** John Kramer, MD personally provided the anesthesia for the case, placing a central venous catheter, non-tunneled in the left internal jugular vein at the beginning of the case (PS II)

**ANESTHESIA:** General endotracheal.

**Anesthesia start time:** 7:45 A.M. **Anesthesia end time:** 10:02 A.M.

**ESTIMATED BLOOD LOSS:** Negligible.

**DESCRIPTION OF PROCEDURE:** The patient was taken to the operative suite and following induction of general anesthesia, we sterilely prepped and draped in routine fashion. A surgical marking pen had been used in the holding area to demarcate our proposed line of the incision around the old eschar. The incision was made in an elliptical fashion around the old eschar and extended on either end about 3 to 4 mm. Small bleeding sites were managed with electrocautery. Dissection was carried through the subcutaneous tissues with electrocautery down to the anterior rectus fascia. At this point, we could palpate the defect measuring about the size of the tip of my finger. We continued to dissect the subcutaneous tissue off the fascia with electrocautery. The hernia was then grasped with Babcock and we incised circumferentially around this. There was a smaller defect just medial. These were combined from one defect which measured about 2-2.5 cm in diameter. The herniated preperitoneal fat was exposed with electrocautery. It was passed off the field to be sent off to pathology. The facial edges were all cleaned back with cautery. They were then reapproximated with interrupted figure-of-eight of #1 Vicryl and a simple #1 Vicryl between the two #1 figure-of-eights. This completed the closure of the fascia without undue tension. The subcutaneous tissues were reapproximated with interrupted 3-0 Vicryl and the skin was approximated with a running subcuticular 4-0 Rapide Vicryl. Dermabond was applied to the incision. The patient was transferred to the recovery room in apparent satisfactory condition.

**GROSS PATHOLOGY:** This is a very pleasant 40-year-old male, whom I had operated on for severe cholecystitis on 01/01/20XX. He developed a bulge in his epigastrium. This indeed showed a defect. There were actually 2 defects but joined together made the total defect measure about 2-2.5 cm in diameter. I did not feel that mesh was necessary on the patient as it approximated without undue tension. There was no other gross pathology noted.

Electronically signed by John Andrews, MD. 1/1/20XX

# CASE 48

## Integumentary system, muscles, and nerves

**Clinical Report Physicians/Mid Levels**
**Memorial Hospital**
**Emergency Department**
**100 East Salt Lake City, UT 80000**
**1/01/20XX 15:19**

**Patient:** SMITH, DUSTIN

**MRN:** W000XXXXX

**Acct#:** W00XXXXX

**INSURANCE:** PRIVATE PAYER, (MEDICARE RULES FOR 65 YRS AND OLDER, External Cause Codes are NOT required)

**Time Seen:** 17:39.

Arrived By private vehicle. Historian patient and family.

**HISTORY OF PRESENT ILLNESS**

Chief Complaint Injury to the right 5th (little) finger. The injury happened just prior to arrival.

He sustained a laceration without damage to the nail. Occurred at work. Was changing a car window today and cut his hand on metal on the car. It bled profusely. The patient is experiencing mild pain.

**REVIEW OF SYSTEMS**

No swelling, tingling, numbness or weakness.

**PAST HISTORY**

Tetanus less than 3 years. Has a "thyroid problem", unsure. The patient's dominant hand is the right.

Tetanus immunization status is up to date.

**Medications:** None.

**Allergies:** No known drug allergies.

**SOCIAL HISTORY**

Nonsmoker.

**ADDITIONAL NOTES**

The nursing notes have been reviewed.

**PHYSICAL EXAM**

**Appearance:** Alert. Oriented X3. No acute distress.

**Vital Signs:** Have been reviewed.

**CVS:** Normal heart rate and rhythm.

**Respiratory:** No respiratory distress.

**Abdomen:** Abdomen soft.

**Extremities:** Right little finger: mild tenderness and subcutaneous 2.5 cm laceration of the dorsal aspect and middle phalanx. Neurovascular intact distally. No damage to the nail or swelling, abrasion,

ecchymosis, puncture wound or deformity. No subungual hematoma or amputation present. No wrist injury.

No hand injury. Extremities are otherwise negative. Neuro, Vascular and Tendons: Vascular status intact. The sensation is intact. Motor intact. Tendon

function intact. No functional tendon deficit or tendon injury seen.

MJ, CRNA personally provided the general endotracheal anesthesia for the case (PS III)

**Anesthesia start time:** 10:00 A.M. **Anesthesia end time:** 10:35 A.M.

Anesthesia was complicated by emergency bleeding of 100 ccs.

**PROGRESS AND PROCEDURES**

Laceration Repair: Location: right little finger. Length: 3 cm. Complexity: simple (local anesthesia used, sutured and closed with tissue adhesive).

Wound depth/shape subcutaneous and involving fascia. Distal neuro/vascular/tendon status normal.

Tendon examined. No tendon deficit. Anesthesia provided using 2% lidocaine. Prepped with Shur Clens.

Wound explored, cleansed and irrigated extensively with normal saline. Closure of superficial layer:

5 0 Prolene (6 sutures). Dressing applied. Splint applied.

**E.D. Course:** 17:43. The patient was seen and examined. Wound cleaned, no tendon injury seen. See wound note. Tetanus up to date. The patient tolerated the procedure well. Good hemostasis.

Patient/family counseled.

**Disposition: Condition:** good. Discharged home. Discharged home in good condition.

**CLINICAL IMPRESSION:**

Laceration to right little finger without damage to the nail.

**INSTRUCTIONS**

Limit use of your hand.

**Warnings: INFECTION:** Watch for signs of infection (increasing heat and redness, pus-like drainage, swelling, or increased pain). Return or see your doctor if these signs occur.

**Prescription Medications:**

Cephalexin 500mg: take 1 tab orally every 6 hours for 7 days. No refills.

**Follow up:**

Return to the emergency department 8 - 10 days for suture removal in two days for a wound check.

Understanding of the discharge instructions verbalized by the patient. Wear splint.

(Electronically signed by Stacy Bank, MD 1/01/20XX 21:11)

Any laboratory data incorporated in this document has been entered by the emergency clinician and may have been summarized or otherwise modified. The original full report is available in Meditech.

**CODING SUMMARY**

**Patient:** Smith, Dustin

**Age/sex:** 29y/M Doctor: Stacy Miller, MD

**INSURANCE:** Private Payer, Medicare rules

**Template:** 09 Hand/Wrist Injury

CASE COMPLEXITY (marked items only)

Clinical **Impression:** Laceration to right little finger

**Symptoms:** Chief Complaint: Injury to the right 5th (little) finger.

**Past History:** dominant hand: Tetanus: NKDA

**Tests and Data:**

Data Score = 0 (Low)

**Procedures:** Laceration Repair E.D. Course

**Disposition:** Condition: good. Discharged home. Discharged home in good condition.

HISTORY AND PHYSICAL SUMMARY (marked items only) H and P Analysis: 3 (does not include medical decision-making considerations).

**HPI:** 3 elements: Severity Context Duration Free Text

**ROS:** 2 elements: Neurologic Musculoskeletal

**PFSH:** 2 elements: Past Hx Social Hx Free Text

Physical Exam Systems: 7 systems: GI CVS Neurologic Respiratory Musculoskeletal Skin

**Constitutional**

Physical Exam Areas: 1 area: Abdomen

**CPT CODE ASSIGNMENTS**

Assigned Level 1 2 3 4 5

**Procedures:** Laceration Repair E.D. Course

**Coder Signature:**______________________________

This is a partial abstract of information documented in the full record. Coder must use independent judgment in selecting codes.

Clinical Report Nurses

**Patient:** SMITH, DUSTIN

**MRN:** W000XXXXX

**Acct#:** W00XXXXXXX

INSURANCE: PRIVATE PAYER, (MEDICARE RULES FOR 65 YRS AND OLDER)

TRIAGE

Initial Assessment

**Acuity:** LEVEL 4.

Alert. No acute distress (Mild distress). 1523 Melcomian, Jen,

**HR:** 67 (regular, normal rate and strong). O2 saturation: 97% room air. 1524 Melcomian, Jen,

**Acuity:** LEVEL 4.

**BP:** 118 / 67 sitting. HR: 56. RR: 18. Temp: 98.5 oral. O2 saturation: 97 % room air. Alert. No acute distress. 1644 Karen Williams, RN.

Medications ("Supposed to take thyroid medicine, but I haven't for about a month and a half."). 1524

Melcomian, Jen

Allergies

No known drug allergies. 1523 Melcomian, Jen

**History**

This occurred just prior to arrival. The patient sustained a laceration from a sharp edge ("Metal on the car."). Pain level now: 6/10. The patient has had numbness and tingling.

PAST HX: No history of diabetes mellitus, hypertension, heart disease or lung disease. No infectious disease exposure. Tetanus status: up to date.

**SOCIAL HX:** Nonsmoker. No alcohol use. No report of abuse.

**Historian:** patient. 1523 Melcomian, Jen, .

Interventions Patient's right 5th finger was wrapped with gauze and secured with tape; Patient provided with a wheelchair to sit in as well. 1525 Melcomian, Jen,

ID band on the patient. To room. 1644 Karen Williams, RN.

**PHYSICAL ASSESSMENT**

Alert. Appears in no acute distress. Oriented X 3. (RT fifth finger, bleeding controlled). Limited ROM present. Capillary refill is less than 2 seconds in the extremities. Extremity pulses are within normal limits. Neurovascular status is intact to the extremity. Normal gait. Skin intact. Skin is warm and dry. 1711 Dee, Christy.

**NURSING PROGRESS NOTES**

1650. Two patient identifiers checked. The plan of care for this patient has been created. Bleeding controlled. Neurovascular extremity check is distal to the injury. Call light placed in reach. Side rails up x 2. Bed placed in the lowest position. Brakes of bed on. 1711 Dee, Christy. Long aluminum foam splint applied to the right little finger by a nurse; distal pulses intact, sensation intact and motor function within normal limits. 1801 Dee, Christy.

**DISPOSITION / DISCHARGE**

Patient reports pain level on departure as 0/10. Condition at departure: improved. Fall risk assessment completed.

No fall risk identified. No learning barriers present. Discharge instructions reviewed with the patient and companion. Reviewed warnings. Reviewed medication. Treatments reviewed. Reviewed referrals. Patient verbalized understanding. Written instructions provided in English. The patient was discharged home and accompanied by a companion. The patient left the Emergency Department ambulatory and via private vehicle. Companion driving. 1802 Dee, Christy.

Locked/Released at 1/01/20XX 18:52 by Dee, Christy,

# CASE 49

# *Femur, open procedures*

**John Andrews, MD**
**Surgery Center**
**1017 Rose Garden Ln.**
**Burley, ID 83768**

**PATIENT:** Thomas Smith

**SEX:** Male

**AGE:** 33

**Medicare-insured**

**DATE OF SERVICE:** 01/01/20XX

**PREOPERATIVE DIAGNOSIS:** Painful hardware x3 of the left ankle.

**POSTOPERATIVE DIAGNOSIS:** Painful hardware x3 of the left ankle.

**PROCEDURE PERFORMED:**

1. Removal of painful hardware x3.
2. Intraoperative x-ray.
3. Application of autogenous Hemocyte tissue graft, left ankle.

**SURGEON:** John Andrews, MD

**ASSISTANT:** None.

**ANESTHESIOLOGIST:** John Kramer, MD personally provided the general endotracheal anesthesia care for the case (PS III)

**ANESTHESIA:** General endotracheal anesthesia.

**Anesthesia start time:** 7:00 A.M. **Anesthesia end time:** 11:47 A.M.

**COMPLICATIONS:** None.

**HEMOSTASIS:** Esmarch to the left calf.

**ESTIMATED BLOOD LOSS:** Approximately 200 mL

**FIXATION MATERIALS:** None.

**SUTURE MATERIALS:** Skin staples.

**INJECTABLES:** 20 mL of 0.5% Marcaine plain.

**BIOLOGICS:** 4 mL of autogenous Hemocyte tissue graft.

**PATHOLOGY SPECIMENS:** Three pieces of internal hardware for the medial and lateral aspect of the left ankle

**DESCRIPTION OF PROCEDURE:** The patient was brought to the operating room and placed on the operating table in the supine position. Following administration of general anesthesia, the left lower extremity was scrubbed, draped and prepped per usual aseptic technique. The left leg was elevated, exsanguinated with an Esmarch bandage which was left in place for a broad expansion to the left calf to maintain hemostasis.

**Procedure #1:** Removal of internal hardware from the medial aspect of the left ankle. Attention was directed to the patient's left ankle. Intraoperative C-arm was introduced to visualize a large 6.5 mm screw within the medial malleolus. A small stab incision was made over the head of the screw and deepened down to deep tissue to reveal a partially exposed head of a Wright Medical 6.5 cannulated screw. Using osteotome and mallet, the bone was broken around the head of the screw and the screw was easily retracted without complication. The wound was flushed with copious amounts of 0.9% normal saline and the skin was closed with skin staples.

**Procedure #2:** Removal of painful hardware from the medial aspect of the left ankle. At this time intraoperative C-arm was used to visualize the second 6.5 mm screw posterior to the first one. The same exact procedure was performed to remove the screw without incident. The closure was done and performed in the same way.

**Procedure #3:** Removal of deep buried hardware from the lateral aspect of the left ankle. At this time attention was directed to the lateral aspect of the left ankle. A previous surgical scare was reopened partially to expose a Wright Medical compression claw plate x2. Through the incision, four screws and two claw plates were removed without incident. The wound was flushed with copious amounts of 0.9% normal saline. The deep tissue was reapproximated and closed with 3-0 Vicryl and the skin was reapproximated and closed with 4-0 Monocryl.

**Procedure #4:** Intraoperative x-ray. At this time intraoperative C-arm was used to visualize the patient's left ankle which was noted to have a very solid fusion with no signs of complication from the hardware removal.

**Procedure #5:** Application of autogenous Hemocyte tissue graft. At this time the patient was injected with 20 mL of 0.5% Marcaine plain for an ankle block. It was then decided to apply an autogenous Hemocyte tissue graft to the lateral aspect of the ankle to facilitate healing due to the deep surgical dissection. 15 mL of blood was drawn from the patient's arm. It was properly centrifuged down to collect the concentrated platelets. Once they were properly harvested and prepared, they were injected percutaneously for a total of 4-5 mL of autogenous Hemocyte tissue graft. The patient was then bandaged with Xeroform, 3 rolls of Kerlix placed in a compression Coban dressing. The tourniquet was released with a good vascular response to the left lower extremity. The patient tolerated the above procedure well and was transported to the recovery room with vital signs stable and intact.

Electronically signed by John Andrews, MD. 1/1/20XX

# CASE 50

# *Bones of the lower leg, ankles, and foot; femoral block*

**John Andrews, MD**
**Surgery Center**
**1017 Rose Garden Ln.**
**Burley, ID 83768**

**PATIENT:** Jane Smith

**SEX:** Female

**AGE:** 69

This is a Commercial Payer (Follow Medicare rules. External causes are NOT required)

**DATE OF SERVICE:** 1/1/20XX

**OPERATIVE REPORT**

**PREOPERATIVE DIAGNOSIS:** Displaced left ankle bimalleolar fracture.

**POSTOPERATIVE DIAGNOSIS:** Displaced left ankle bimalleolar fracture.

**PROCEDURE PERFORMED:** Open treatment with internal fixation of the left ankle bimalleolar fracture.

**SURGEON:** John Andrews, MD

**ASSISTANT:** John Kramer, MD

**ANESTHESIOLOGIST:** John Thompson, MD personally provided the general endotracheal anesthesia with a left femoral block for the case while directing 3 CRNAs (PS III). JT, MD placed a central venous catheter in the left internal jugular vein at the beginning of the case.

**CRNAs:** JJ, CRNA, MG, CRNA, LL, CRNA

**ANESTHESIA:** General endotracheal with a left femoral nerve block.

**Anesthesia start time:** 9:00 A.M. **Anesthesia end time:** 11:57 A.M.

**COMPLICATIONS:** None.

**ESTIMATED BLOOD LOSS:** 50 mL.

**TOURNIQUET TIME:** 88 minutes at 300 mmHg.

**SPECIMENS:** None.

**FINDINGS:** Left ankle bimalleolar fracture

**IMPLANTS:** Synthes locking one-third tubular plate, with 2 individual 4.0 mm cannulated screws, a 3.5 mm shaft screw, two individual 4.0 mm cancellous screws, a 3.5 mm cortex screw and four individual 3.5 mm locking screws.

**INDICATIONS:** This is a 69-year-old female who sustained a left ankle fracture 3 days ago after running a marathon. She was initially placed into a splint and referred to the office. She was found to have a left ankle bimalleolar fracture. The diagnosis, treatment options, risks, and benefits were discussed with the patient. Because of the displaced nature of the left ankle bimalleolar fracture, it was recommended to proceed with open treatment with internal fixation of the left ankle bimalleolar fracture. This would allow for reduction of the fracture back to a more anatomic position, with internal fixation and stabilization to provide for stability of the ankle. The details of the procedure were discussed with the patient using lay terms to the best of my ability, including the risks and benefits and expected outcomes. The risks of the procedure include, but are not limited to: bleeding, infection, blood clot, pain, swelling, numbness, stiffness, or arthritis of the ankle. The risks also include injury to blood vessels, nerves, ligaments, tendons, muscle, cartilage, or bone of the ankle. The risks also include injury to blood vessels, nerves, ligaments, tendons, muscle, cartilage, or bone of the ankle. The risks also include injury to blood vessels, nerves, ligaments, tendons, muscle, cartilage or bone of the ankle. The risks also include foot-drop or deformity of the ankle, fracture nonunion, fracture malunion, hardware irritation requiring removal or the need for additional left ankle surgery. The patient verbalized understanding of this and gave her informed written consent.

**DESCRIPTION OF PROCEDURE:** The patient was taken to the operative suite under the guidance of anesthesia and placed in the supine position on the operating table. After appropriate general anesthesia had been given, a tourniquet was placed high on the left thigh. The left lower extremity was sterilely prepped and draped in the usual sterile fashion. The left lower extremity was exsanguinated and the tourniquet was inflated to 300 mmHg.

A longitudinal incision was made over the lateral aspect of the left ankle distal fibula lateral malleolar fracture. This was found to be a long oblique fracture. This fracture did extend down to the distal tibia/fibula articulation. Careful sharp and blunt dissection was carried through the subcutaneous tissues over the lateral malleolus, with electrocautery used as needed to help achieve hemostasis. The deep fascial tissue was incised in a longitudinal fashion and carefully retracted. The periosteum over the fracture was minimally elevated. This allowed for visualization of the left ankle distal fibula fracture. This was a long oblique fracture, with a slight amount of comminution noted. The fracture was irrigated and debrided. A bone reduction clamp was used to help reduce the fracture back to a more anatomic position. The position of this fracture was checked with both AP, mortise and lateral view x-rays. The fracture of the distal fibula was found to be reduced to a near anatomic position.

Initial stabilization was achieved by placing a 3.5 mm shaft screw across the fracture from anterior to posterior. This was done in the standard technique of drilling both cortices measuring and placing the appropriate length 3.5 mm shaft screw. This provided good initial stabilization. A second shaft screw was also placed in the same technique, proximal to the first. This also achieved good initial stabilization.

Attention was then turned to definitive fixation using a locking one-third tubular plate. This was contoured along the lateral aspect of the distal fibula. The plate was initially secured to the distal fibula proximal to the long oblique fracture. This was done by placing a 3.5 mm cortex screw proximal to the fracture. This was done in the standard technique of drilling both cortices, measuring and placing the appropriate length 3.5 mm cortex screw through the plate, achieving good bicortical fixation. Three additional 3.5 mm locking screws were able to be placed proximal to the fracture. These were done in the standard technique or drilling both cortices, measuring and placing the appropriate length 3.5 mm locking screw. Once again these were placed proximal to the long oblique fracture.

The remaining portion of the fracture was then bridged to avoid injury to this portion of the fracture. Therefore, three additional screws were placed distal to the fracture. These were done in the standard technique of drilling one cortex, measuring and placing the appropriate length 4.0 mm cancellous screw on two occasions and a 3.5 mm locking screw as well. These achieved good stabilization distal to the fracture.

The clamp was removed from the distal fibula. The proximal shaft screw was also removed as it was providing minimal stabilization at this point.

C-arm fluoroscopy verified in the AP, the mortise and the lateral views that the distal fibula fracture had been reduced to a near anatomic position. There was good stabilization provided with good fixation noted.

A Cotton stress test was then performed to check the syndesmosis. The syndesmosis was found to be stable to stress testing.

Attention was then turned to fixation of the medial malleolus. A longitudinal incision was made over the medial malleolus. Careful sharp and blunt dissection was carried through the subcutaneous tissues with electrocautery used as needed to help achieve hemostasis. The medial malleolus fracture was identified. Minimal periosteal elevation was performed. The wound was irrigated and debrided. A bone reduction clamp was used to help reduce the fracture back to a near anatomic position. Small amounts of comminution were noted at the fracture. These very small comminuted fracture fragments were able to be removed.

Once the fracture was reduced, C-arm fluoroscopy verified in the AP, the mortise and the lateral views that the fracture had been reduced to a near anatomic position. Two initial guidewires were placed across the fracture from distal to proximal. These were measured and the appropriate length 5.0 mm partially-threaded cannulated screws were placed over each of these guidewires, advancing from distal to proximal across the medial malleolus fracture. These achieved good fixation. The guidewires were removed from the medial malleolus.

C-arm fluoroscopy verified in AP, the lateral and the mortise views that the medial malleolus fracture was also reduced to a near anatomic position, with good fixation noted. There also appeared to be on the lateral view x-ray the possibility of a very small posterior malleolus fracture fragment. This did not involve the articular surface. Therefore no additional treatment was necessary for this nondisplaced posterior malleolus fracture.

C-arm fluoroscopy verified in the AP, the mortise and the lateral views that the bimalleolar fractures had been reduced to a near anatomic position. There was a good fixation with the hardware with good position of the fractures.

The tourniquet was deflated. Electrocautery was used as needed to help achieve hemostasis. The wounds were thoroughly irrigated using copious amounts of normal saline. The deep fascial tissue was approximated using #1 Vicryl. The subcutaneous tissues were approximated using 2-0 Vicryl. The skin edges were approximated using 3-0 nylon. A sterile dressing was applied to the patient's left ankle, followed by the placement of a very well padded left ankle posterior splint with stirrups.

All instrument, needle and sponge counts were correct. The anesthesiologist then performed a left lower extremity femoral nerve block. The patient tolerated the procedure well and was transported to the postanesthesia care unit under the guidance of anesthesia in stable and satisfactory condition.

Electronically signed by John Andrews, MD. 1//20XX

**John Andrews, MD**

**Surgery Center**

**1017 Rose Garden Ln.**

**Burley, ID 83768**

**PATIENT:** Jane Smith

**SEX:** Female

**AGE:** 69

This is a Commercial Payer (Follow Medicare rules. External causes are NOT required)

**DATE OF SERVICE:** 1/1/20XX

**HISTORY AND PHYSICAL**

**CHIEF COMPLAINT:** Left ankle pain.

**HISTORY OF PRESENT ILLNESS:** A 69-year-old female with left ankle pain after running a marathon since 06/15/20XX.

**PAST MEDICAL HISTORY:** Unremarkable, dental surgery.

**SOCIAL HISTORY:** Tobacco.

**MEDICATIONS:** Noncontributory.

**PHYSICAL EXAMINATION:**

**GENERAL:** Within normal limits.

**HEART:** Within normal limits.

**LUNGS:** Normal breath sounds.

**EXTREMITIES:** Left ankle fracture TTP.

**PELVIC:** Deferred.

**HEENT:** Within normal limits.

**NECK:** Within normal limits.

**NEUROLOGIC:** Distally NVI.

**SKIN:** Within normal limits.

**BREASTS:** Deferred.

**ABDOMEN:** Within normal limits.

**VASCULAR:** Within normal limits.

**LYMPHATIC:** Within normal limits.

**PSYCHIATRIC:** Within normal limits.

**DIAGNOSTIC DATA:** X-rays show left ankle bimalleolar fracture.

**IMPRESSION:** Left ankle bimalleolar fracture.

**PLAN:** ORIF left ankle bimalleolar fracture.

Electronically signed by John Andrews, MD. 1/1/20XX

# Solutions

## 1.

### Codes

L89.153, G93.1, V80.711, Y92.828, Y99.8, Z93.0, Z93.1, 44320

### Overall anesthesiology code for the case for the billing anesthesiologist

00790-QK-P3, 36556

### Overall anesthesiology code for the case for the billing CRNA

00790-QX-P3, 36556

00790 Anesthesia for intraperitoneal procedures in upper abdomen including laparoscopy, not otherwise specified

**ASA Crosswalk Lookup:** CPT code= Base value units= Anesthesia code

44320= 7 base value units= 00790

36556= 4 base units= 00532

### Units calculation

Total Units=Base+Time+Physical Status+Emergency=7+12.68+1.0+0=-20.68

### Clinical viewpoint

The patient had a stage III decubitus ulcer (L89.153) which was a full-thickness skin loss ulcer involving necrosis of the subcutaneous tissue. A decubitus ulcer is a pressure ulcer. The patient has severe systemic disease that is not a constant threat to life (PS III) including anoxic brain injury from falling off a horse in leisure (V80.711, Y92.828, Y99.8) and a stage III sacral decubitus ulcer with a tracheostomy (Z93.0) and gastrostomy (Z93.1) already in place as status-post. The patient received a sigmoid colostomy (44320) for fecal diversion to help the healing of this wound that may have the possibility that that wound would not heal. One CRNA placed a non-tunneled central venous catheter into the internal jugular vein (36556), which counts as an anesthesia code for both the billing anesthesiologist and CRNA. The overall anesthesia code for the case is 00790 (base value units=7) for anesthesia for intraperitoneal procedures in upper abdomen including laparoscopy. The anesthesia time for this case began at the instillation of general endotracheal anesthesia and ended with the anesthesiologist and CRNAs treating the patient in the post-anesthesia care unit.

## 2.

### Codes

L92.9, 46270, 46600-59

### ASA Crosswalk Lookup

46270=5 base value units=00902

46600=4 base value units=00811

### Overall anesthesiology code for the billing anesthesiologist

00902-QK-P3, +99135

00902 Anesthesia for; anorectal procedure

### Units calculation

Total Units=Base+Time+Physical status+Emergency=5+4.33+1+5=15.3 (Can round up or down for exam)

Relative value units

46270=11.37 RVU

46600=1.18 RVU

### Clinical viewpoint

The patient has excessive granulation tissue in a sinus tract as a remnant of a previously excised pilonidal cyst, which can be found in the ICD-10-CM medical codebook as a granulomatous disorder of the skin and subcutaneous tissue (L92.9). A pilonidal cyst is an abscess near the natal cleft of the buttock which is also referred to as a pilonidal sinus or sacrococcygeal fistula. The patient underwent diagnostic anoscopy (46600) and surgical treatment of anal fistula (fistulectomy/fistulotomy); subcutaneous (46270). The CPT codes are in correct relative value order (46600 relative value units=1.19, 46260 RVU=11.31). The patient has a severe systemic disease (PS III). The anesthesia was for an anorectal procedure (00902) and the anesthesiologist conducted the general endotracheal anesthesia while concurrently directing three other procedures (HCPCS Level II modifier QK). The two procedures 46600 and 46270 are not normally reported together (modifier 59).

## 3.

### Codes

Z46.59, Z90.49, 43275

### Overall anesthesiology code for the case for the billing anesthesiologist

00732-QY-P3

### Overall anesthesiology code for the case for the billing CRNA

00732-QX-P3

00732 Anesthesia for upper gastrointestinal endoscopic procedures, endoscope introduced proximal to duodenum; endoscopic retrograde cholangiopancreatography (ERCP)

Units calculation=Base+Time+Physical status+Emergency=6+4.4+1+0=11.4

### Clinical viewpoint

The patient underwent a procedure for removal of stents from biliary ducts utilizing endoscopic retrograde cholangiopancreatography (ERCP) (CPT 43275). The encounter is for fitting and adjustment of other gastrointestinal appliance and device (Z46.59) and the patient is status post cholecystectomy which is medically coded in ICD-10-CM as an acquired absence of other specified parts of the digestive tract (Z90.49). A cystic bile duct leak for which the cholecystectomy was originally performed is systemic medical illness (PS III). The anesthesia is for upper gastrointestinal endoscopic procedures, endoscope introduced proximal to duodenum; ERCP (00732). The HCPCS II modifiers are QY Medical direction of one certified registered nurse anesthetist (CRNA) by an anesthesiologist for the billing anesthesiologist and QX CRNA service: with medical direction by a physician.

## 4.

### Codes

K40.20, L72.3, K91.61, 49505-50, 11402-59

### ASA Crosswalk Lookup

49505=4 base value units=00830

11402=3 base value units=00400

### Relative value units for relative value order

49505=15.07 RVU

11402=3.29 RVU

### Overall anesthesiology code for the billing CRNA

00830-QZ-QS-P2, +99140

00830 Anesthesia for hernia repairs in the lower abdomen; not otherwise specified

Units calculation=Base+Time+Physical status+Emergency= 4+8.6+0+2.0=14.6 (Can round either up or down for CANPC exam)

### Clinical viewpoint

The patient has bilateral direct inguinal hernias (K40.20) and a small sebaceous cyst (L72.3) of the left groin. The patient underwent open bilateral inguinal hernia repair, age 5 years or older; reducible (49505-50) and excision of a benign lesion or 1.0 cm sebaceous cyst from left groin which is on the left upper thigh with 0.5 cm margins or a total excised diameter of 2.0 cm (11402-59). The procedure on a digestive system structure (hernia) was complicated by intra-operative hemorrhage (K91.61). The two procedures are performed in the same operative session and not normally reported together (modifier 59). The bilateral direct inguinal hernias combined with a small sebaceous cyst of the groin can be considered to be mild systemic illness (P2). The ASA Crosswalk determines that 49505 corresponds to a higher base value unit value than 11402; therefore, the overall anesthesiology code for the case is 00830 Anesthesia for hernia repairs; not otherwise specified. The anesthesia service is monitored anesthesia care (QS). The anesthesia was complicated by emergency bleeding of 500 cc's blood loss from the bilateral direct inguinal hernia repairs, corresponding to a qualifying circumstances code of +99140.

## 5.

### Codes

C50.411, Z17.0, 19301, 19125-59, 38525, 88307, 88331

### Relative value units

19301=18.86 RVU

19125=18.46 RVU

38525=12.64 RVu

### Overall anesthesiology code for the case for the billing anesthesiologist

01610-AD-P4, 36620

01610 Anesthesia for all procedures on nerves, muscles, tendons, fascia, and bursae of shoulder and axilla

Units calculation=Base+Time+Physical status+Emergency= 5+14.4+2+0=21.4

### Clinical viewpoint

The patient has estrogen-receptor (+) (Z17.0) breast cancer of the right upper outer quadrant (C50.411) for which she undergoes a right lumpectomy or partial mastectomy (19301) with needle localization or placement of a radiological marker (19125) and sentinel node biopsy (38525). A breast mastectomy specimen-partial (88307) and a single specimen of a first tissue block with a frozen section during pathology consultation during surgery (88331) were obtained. The general endotracheal anesthesia is for all procedures on nerves, muscles, tendons, fascia, and bursae of shoulder and axilla (01610). A radial arterial catheter (36620) was placed at the beginning of the case by the anesthesiologist; therefore, 36620 counts in the overall anesthesiology code for the case. The anesthesiologist performed the anesthesia for the case while running five procedures concurrently (HCPCS II modifier AD).

## 6.

### Codes

C18.4, 44204

### Overall anesthesiology code for the case for the billing anesthesiologist

00790-QY-P4, +99140, 36556

### Overall anesthesiology code for the case for the billing CRNA

00790-QX-P4, +99140, 36556

00790 Anesthesia for intraperitoneal procedures in upper abdomen including laparoscopy; not otherwise specified

+99140 Anesthesia complicated by emergency conditions

Units calculation=Base+Time+Physical status+Emergency=7+13.8+2+2=24.8 (Can round up or down for CANPC exam)

### Clinical viewpoint

The patient has adenocarcinoma of the transverse colon, with no noted metastases (C18.4). The patient underwent a transverse colectomy for removal of the adenocarcinoma. The treatment is for active intestinal cancer. For this case, there is only one CPT code. Therefore, the CPT code 44204 corresponds to the anesthesia code 00790, looking up the code in ASA Crosswalk. The anesthesiologist placed the non-tunneled central venous catheter (36556) in this patient, and therefore the CPT code counts for the case for the billing anesthesiology staff. The surgery was complicated by emergency bleeding (+99140) and therefore added 2 base value units to the units calculation (Units=24.8).

## 7.

J93.83, 32551

### Overall anesthesiology code for the case for the billing anesthesiologist

99156, +99157

99156 Moderate sedation services provided by a physician or other qualified health care professional other than the physician or other qualified health care professional performing the diagnostic or therapeutic service that the sedation support; initial 15 minutes intra-service time, patient age 5 years or older

+99157 each additional 15 minutes intra-service time

### Clinical viewpoint

Versed (midazolam) is a benzodiazepine used for moderate conscious sedation in this anesthesiology case. Moderate conscious sedation is a drug-induced depression of consciousness during which patients respond purposefully to verbal commands, either alone or accompied by light tactile stimulation. The moderate sedation service (99156, +99157) was provided by the anesthesiologist for 32 minutes, which is different from the doctor who performed the thoracostomy (32551). For each additional 15 minutes, the number of minutes has to be a minimum of 8 minutes to count as an additional 15 minutes intra-service time.

## 8.

### Codes

C16.1, D49.0, 47100-51, 59, 49000, 88305

### Overall anesthesiology code for the case for the billing anesthesiologist

00790-QK-P4, 93503, +99140, +99135, +99100

### Overall anesthesiology for the case for the billing CRNA

00790-QX-P4, 93503, +99140, +99135, +99100

00790 Anesthesia for intraperitoneal procedures in upper abdomen including laparoscopy; not otherwise specified

+99100 Anesthesia for a patient of extreme age, younger than 1 year and older than 70

+99135 Anesthesia complicated by utilization of controlled hypotension

+99140 Anesthesia complicated by emergency conditions

Units calculation=Base+Time+Physical status+Emergency=7+11.33+2+8=28.3 (Can round up or down for CANPC exam)

Units calculation if the patient were a Medicare patient=Base+Time=7+11.33=18.3 (Can round up or down for CANPC exam)

## Clinical viewpoint

The patient had carcinoma of the fundus of the stomach (C16.1) and small tumors were noted in the left lobe of the liver upon laparotomy. Exploratory laparotomy of the abdomen (49000) was performed with a wedge biopsy of the liver (47100-51, 59). Part of one lymph node (88305) from the liver was removed and sent to pathology for analysis. Anesthesia was for intraperitoneal procedures in the upper abdomen (00790). A Swan—Ganz catheter (+93503) was placed at the beginning of the case for monitoring purposes. Since the anesthesiologist placed the Swan-Ganz catheter, the CPT code counts for anesthesia billing purposes. If the surgeon placed the Swan-Ganz catheter, the CPT code for the Swan-Ganz catheter would not be included in the CPT coding for the case for the anesthesia. The patient was over 70 years of age (+99140) and the anesthesia was complicated by the utilization of controlled hypotension (+99135). Therefore, there were two qualifying circumstances for the case which were factors in the units calculation. The anesthesiologist was directing two concurrent anesthesia procedures (HCPCS II modifier QK). In the actual CANPC exam, the terminology 2 or more CRNAs is used corresponding to two or more concurrent procedures as stated in HCPCS II. The CPT codes for the case are in correct relative value order.

## 9.

## Codes

K22.2, Z90.49, 43245

## Overall anesthesiology code for the case for the billing anesthesiologist

00731-QY-P4

## Overall anesthesiology code for the case for the billing CRNA

00731-QX-P4

Units calculation=Base+Time+Physical status+Emergency=5+4.13+2+0=11.13 (Can round either up or down for CANPC exam)

00731 Anesthesia for upper gastrointestinal endoscopic procedures, endoscope introduced proximal to duodenum; not otherwise specified

## Clinical viewpoint

The patient had an esophageal stricture (K22.2) causing dysphagia. The patient had an esophagogastroduodenoscopy, flexible, transoral performed with dilation of gastric/duodenal stricture (s) (43245). The patient also had a history of an Ivor-Lewis resection for adenocarcinoma (PS IV). The adenocarcinoma is not defined but the procedure is not for the adenocarcinoma and therefore the diagnosis is irrelevant for the service. The anesthesia (00731) is for upper gastrointestinal endoscopic procedures, endoscope introduced proximal to the duodenum. The surgeon placed the central venous catheter. Therefore, the CPT code 36556 is not included in the overall anesthesiology code for the case. The anesthesiologist or CRNA has to place the central venous catheter, radial arterial catheter, Swan-Ganz catheter, or transesophageal echocardiogram at the beginning of the case for the CPT codes for these procedures to count for the overall anesthesiology code for the case.

## 10.

### Codes

C50.912, C77.3, 36561, +77001-59, 71046

### Overall anesthesiology code for the case for the billing anesthesiologist

00532-QK-P4, +99100

Units calculation=Base+Time+Physical status+Emergency=4+4.33+2+1=11.33

00532 Anesthesia for access to the central venous circulation

### Clinical viewpoint

The patient has left breast cancer (C50.912) with metastatic disease to left axillary lymph nodes (C77.3). A Port-a-Cath which is a central venous catheter with a port (36561) was placed under fluoroscopic guidance for central venous access in order to instill chemotherapy. The patient is over 70 years old, and therefore the patient has a qualifying circumstance or what I term Emergency of +99100. The anesthesiologist personally performed the general endotracheal anesthesia for the case (modifier QK).

## 11.

### Codes

I51.81, E03.9, 93452, 93307-51, 99283, 99291, 93000

### Overall anesthesiology code for the case for the billing anesthesiologist

01920-QK-P3, 93312, 93503

### Overall anesthesiology code for the case for the billing CRNA

01920-QX-P3, 93312, 93503

01920 Anesthesia for cardiac catheterization including coronary angiography and ventriculography

### Relative value units (RVU) in relative value order

93452=17.69 RVU

93307=3.97 RVU

99283=3.32 RVU

99291=3.15 RVU

93000=0.24 RVU

### Units calculation

Total units=Base+Time+Physical status+Emergency=7+12.87+1+0=20.87

## Clinical viewpoint

The patient visited the Emergency Department (99283) with chest pain and underwent an EKG (93000), which showed ST-T changes suggestive of myocardial ischemia and a transesophageal echocardiogram (93307), which showed a regional wall motion abnormality in the apex of the left ventricle, which corroborated the presence of myocardial ischemia. The patient underwent left heart catheterization including intraprocedural injection(s) for left ventriculography, imaging supervision, and interpretation, when performed (93452), which found Takotsubo cardiomyopathy (I51.81). The anesthesia (01920) was for cardiac catheterization including coronary angiography and ventriculography. The patient had cardiomyopathy and hypothyroidism and therefore had a physical status modifier P3 for a patient with the severe systemic disease. The anesthesiologist placed a Swan Ganz catheter or flow-directed catheter for monitoring purposes (93503) and performed a TEE (93312) at the beginning of the case. Because the anesthesiologist placed the Swan Ganz catheter and performed the TEE, the CPT codes count for the overall anesthesiology code for the case.

# 12.

## Codes

I27.0, 93451, 78580, 99291, 78579, +99292, 76827, 36600, 93000

## Overall anesthesiology code for the case for the billing anesthesiologist

01920-AA-P3

01920 Anesthesia for cardiac catheterization including coronary angiography and ventriculography

## Units calculation

Total units=Base+Time+Physical status+Emergency=7+11.33+1+0=19.33

## Clinical viewpoint

The patient was admitted into the telemetry unit of critical care (99291, +99292) for 105 minutes for idiopathic primary pulmonary hypertension (127.0) until the patient underwent right heart catheterization in the critical care unit (99291, +99292). The patient underwent ventilation-perfusion scan imaging, which involved pulmonary perfusion imaging (78580) and pulmonary ventilation imaging (78579) and Doppler echocardiography (76827). An EKG (93000) was performed. Arterial puncture (36600) was performed for arterial blood gas analysis. The anesthesia (01920) was for cardiac catheterization including coronary angiography and ventriculography.

# 13.

## Codes

I21.09, I10, D64.9, 99291, 99223, +99292, 92977

## Overall anesthesiology code for the case

99291, +99292 x 2

Anesthesia cares not typically required.

### Clinical viewpoint

The patient had an ST elevation (STEMI) myocardial infarction (I21.09) involving other coronary artery of anterior wall (anteroseptal), which is high complexity in medical decision making and implies a comprehensive history and a comprehensive physical exam in a dangerous, urgent situation. The patient was treated with coronary thrombolytic therapy utilizing streptokinase infusion (92977) in which anesthesia care is not typically required according to the ASA Crosswalk. The patient received two hours of treatment in the critical care unit (99291, +99292 x 2), which includes services typically performed in the critical care unit which are likely in this case, including cardiac output measurements, chest x-rays, pulse oximetry, blood gases, ECGs, blood pressures, hematologic data, ventilatory management, and vascular access procedures. A vascular access procedure is necessary for the thrombolytic infusion with streptokinase. The patient is admitted to the inpatient hospital University Medical Center after leaving from the CCU (99223). All of the ICD-10-CM diagnoses are present on admission (POA=Y).

## 14.

### Codes

K25.9, K29.80, K29.60, K44.9, K21.9, I10, 43235

### Overall anesthesiology code for the case for the billing anesthesiologist

99156, +99157

### Clinical viewpoint

The patient underwent anesthesia of moderate (conscious) sedation with Versed for the esophagogastroduodenoscopy (43235). The moderate sedation was performed by the physician, which in this case was the anesthesiologist other than the physician or surgeon performing the diagnostic service for a time of 27 minutes (99156, +99157). 8 minutes additional from 15 minutes intra-service time is mandatory to code +99157, which in this case is 12 minutes beyond the initial 15 minutes (99156).

## 15.

### Codes

S42.451A, I10, E10.9, 24575

### ASA Crosswalk Lookup

24575=4 base units=01740

### Overall anesthesiology code for the billing CRNA

01740-QZ-P3

Units calculation= Base+Time+Physical status modifier+Emergency=

4+11.6+1+0=16.6

### Clinical viewpoint

The patient has been treated for a displaced comminuted fracture of the right elbow with an open treatment of humeral epicondylar fracture, medial or lateral, including internal fixation, which was performed (24575). The anesthesia was for open or surgical arthroscopic procedures of the elbow (01740). The CRNA performed the general endotracheal anesthesia by himself without the help of an anesthesiologist (HCPCS II modifier QZ).

## 16.

### Codes

S62.631B, M96.810, X58.XXXA, Y92.63, Y93.79, Y93.G1, Y99.0, 26765-F1

### ASA Crosswalk Lookup

26765=3 base value units=01830

### Overall anesthesiology code for the billing anesthesiologist

01830-AD-P2, +99140

### Overall anesthesiology code for the billing CRNA

01830-QX-P2, +99140

Units calculation=Base+Time+Physical status+Emergency=3.0+9.47+0+2=14.47

### Clinical viewpoint

The patient had an accident by catching his hand in a food-processing machine at work in a factory (ICD-10-CM codes X58.XXXA, Y92.63, Y93.79, Y93.G1, Y99.0). The open fracture of the distal phalanx of his index finger of the left hand (S62.631B) required open treatment (26765-F1). The anesthesia (01830) was for open or surgical arthroscopic/endoscopic procedures on distal radius, distal ulna, wrist, or hand joints; not otherwise specified. There was an emergency condition (+99140) of emergency hemorrhage complicating the orthopedic surgery (M96.810). The time units are 9.47 (142 minutes/15).

## 17.

### Codes

I25.10, 33533, +33519, +33508

### Relative value units

33533 (54.09)

+33519 (15.78)

+33508 (0.47)

### ASA Crosswalk Lookup

33533=18 base value units=00567

+33519=not a primary procedure code

+33508=not a primary procedure code

### Overall anesthesiology code for the billing anesthesiologist

00567-QK-P3

### Overall anesthesiology code for the billing CRNA

00567-QX-P3

Units calculation=Base+Time+Physical status+Emergency=18+22.80+1.0+0=41.80

### Clinical viewpoint

The patient had severe coronary artery disease (I25.10) treated by quadruple coronary bypass surgery involving single arterial graft (33533) of the left internal mammary artery (LIMA) to the left anterior descending artery. Additional procedures include combined arterial-venous grafting with 3 venous grafts (+33519) of the saphenous vein graft to the obtuse marginal, diagonal artery and posterior descending artery. Surgical endoscopy was performed for the video-assisted harvest of veins for coronary artery bypass procedure (+33508). The CPT codes are in relative value order. The anesthesia (00567) was for direct coronary artery bypass grafting with pump oxygenator as in cardiopulmonary bypass.

## 18.

### Codes

O44.13, O60.14X1, O60.14X2, O30.043, D62, O99.02, Z37.2, Z3A.33, 59510

### ASA Crosswalk Lookup

59510=7 base value units=01961

### Overall anesthesiology code for the billing anesthesiologist

01961-AA-P3, +99140

Units calculation= Base+Time+Physical status+Emergency=7.0+20.20+1.0+2.0=30.2

### Clinical viewpoint

The patient had complete placenta previa with hemorrhage (O44.13) with the preterm delivery of twins (O60.14X1, O60.14X2, O30.043). Acute post-hemorrhagic anemia complicated the childbirth (D62, O99.02). The patient underwent primary low cesarean delivery of twins (59510). The anesthesia was for cesarean delivery only (01961). In this case, the anesthesia was complicated by emergency conditions (+99140), which was the hemorrhage during the cesarean section.

## 19.

### Codes

D66, D62, 96413, 36569, 36430-59, J7190

### ASA Crosswalk Lookup

96413=4 base units value=00532

36569=4 base units value=00532

36430=anesthesia code does not exist

### Relative value units

36569=9.56 RVU

36430=1.46 RVU

J7190= 0 RVU

### Overall anesthesiology code for the case for the billing anesthesiologist

00532-QK-P3, +99135

### Overall anesthesiology code for the case for the billing CRNA

00532-QX-P3, +99135

### Units calculation

Units=Base+Time+Physical status+Emergency=5.0+3.8+1.0+5.0=14.8

If the patient were a Medicare patient,

Units calculation=Base+Time=5.0+3.8=8.8

Clinical viewpointA peripherally inserted central venous catheter (PICC) (36569) was placed for transfusion of 4 units of packed red blood cells (36430) and an infusion of clotting factors for hemophilia (D66). The patient presents with acute posthemorrhagic anemia (D62). Factor VIII is the clotting factor used to treat hemophilia with an infusion in this case (J7190). According to field avoidance theory, a patient in a prone position has a minimum base value unit=5. In this case, the anesthesia code for the case has a base value unit=4. For the units calculations, the base value unit=5.0 according to field avoidance theory. The anesthesia (+99135) was complicated by controlled hypotension for 25 minutes during the case. In my units calculation, the general word Emergency refers to Qualifying circumstances.

## 20.

### Codes

D24.1, 19101

### Overall anesthesiology for the case for the billing anesthesiologist

00400-AD-P2, +99140

### Overall anesthesiology code for the case for the billing CRNA

00400-QX-P2, +99140

### Units calculation

Units calculation=Base+Time+Physical status+Emergency=3.0+2.33+0+2.0=7.33

### Clinical viewpoint

The patient has a right breast fibroadenoma (D24.1) treated by excisional breast biopsy (19101). The anesthesia (0400) is for procedures on the integumentary system on the extremities, anterior trunk, and perineum. The anesthesia was complicated by the emergency condition of emergency bleeding (+99140).

## 21.

### Codes

C78.02, Z85.828, Z90.5, 32505

### Overall anesthesiology code for the case for the billing anesthesiologist

00541-QS-QY-P4

### Overall anesthesiology code for the case for the billing CRNA

00541-QS-QX-P4

Units calculation=Base+Time+Physical status+Emergency=15.0+11.47+2.0+0.0=28.47 (Can round up to 25 or down to 24 for CANPC exam)

### Clinical viewpoint

The patient underwent left thoracotomy with wedge excision of his left upper lobe mass (32505) from metastatic renal carcinoma to the lung (C78.02). The patient has a right nephrectomy (Z90.5)-treated carcinoma of the kidney (Z85.828). The anesthesia is for thoracotomy procedures involving lungs, pleura, diaphragm, and mediastinum (including surgical thoracoscopy); utilizing one-lung ventilation. Although not stated, the procedure utilized one-lung ventilation, as determined by the anesthesia code. The anesthesiology code can often delineate more information. For example, the anesthesia code 00567 means that the anesthesia for direct coronary artery bypass grafting was performed with pump oxygenator, even if the information is not stated in the body text of the case. The anesthesia was a monitored anesthesia care service (modifier QS). The moribund patient has carcinoma and is therefore not expected to survive without the operation (PS IV).

## 22.

### Codes

K62.3, K62.1, K57.30, K52.9, R19.4, 45380

### Overall anesthesiology code for the case

99152, +99153

### Clinical viewpoint

The patient had rectal polyps (K62.1) with rectal prolapse (K62.3) and significant sigmoid diverticulosis (K57.30) and unspecified colitis (K52.9) with a change in bowel habits (R19.4). Colonoscopy (45380) was performed with a biopsy of two of the polyps with cold biopsy forceps. Moderate sedation services (99152, +99153) were provided by the same physician, the surgeon or other qualified health care professional performing the diagnostic or therapeutic service that the sedation supports, requiring the presence of an independent trained observer, the R.N. to assist in the monitoring of the patient's level of consciousness and physiological status. The moderate sedation was for 25 minutes as greater than 8/15 minutes counts as the add-on code (+99153) in this case.

## 23.

### Codes

G54.6, Z89.511, C40.21, Z85.830, Z92.21, 0230T

### ASA Crosswalk Lookup

0230T Anesthesia care not typically required

### Clinical viewpoint

The patient had a phantom limb syndrome with pain (G54.6). Phantom limb pain occurs when nerves are re-wired by the spinal cord and brain following amputation of the same extremity. The patient has a right below-the-knee amputation (Z89.511). The patient underwent injection of an anesthetic (Marcaine), transforaminal epidural in the L2 spinal space (0230T) as a right sympathetic lumbar block. Injection of an anesthetic is the nerve block as the anesthesia for this case. Please note that right sympathetic lumbar block is the treatment for phantom limb pain syndrome. As noted in the ASA Crosswalk, anesthesia care is not typically required for 0230T.

## 24.

### Codes

C91.00, 38220

### ASA Crosswalk Lookup

38220=5 base value units=01112

### Overall anesthesiology code for the case for the billing anesthesiologist

01112-QK-P4

### Overall anesthesiology code for the case for the billing CRNA

01112-QX-P4

Units calculation=Base+Time+Physical status+Emergency=5.0+5.80+2.0+0=12.8 (Can round up or down for CANPC exam)

### Clinical viewpoint

The patient underwent diagnostic bone marrow aspiration of the sternum (38220) to diagnose acute lymphocytic leukemia (C91.00). The patient has a severe systemic disease (cancer) that is a constant threat to life (PS IV). The patient underwent anesthesia for bone marrow aspiration and/or biopsy, anterior or posterior iliac crest (38220).

## 25.

### Codes

C61, 36556

### Overall anesthesia code for the case for the billing anesthesiologist

00532-AA-P4, +99100

Units calculation=Base=Time+Physical status+Emergency=4.0+3.67+2.0+1.0=10.7 (Can round up or down for actual CANPC exam)

### Clinical viewpoint

The elderly 74-year-old patient with prostate carcinoma (C61) underwent insertion of a percutaneous subclavian venous catheter (non-tunneled by default) (36556) by prepping the right upper chest. The patient has a malignant neoplasm of the prostate (PS IV) and has a qualifying circumstance or what I term Emergency of anesthesia for a patient of extreme age, younger than 1 year and older than 70 (+99100). The anesthesia is for access for central venous circulation. The access for central venous circulation, in this case, is required for the treatment of his prostate carcinoma.

## 26.

### Codes

12031, 11402, D36.14

### ASA Crosswalk Lookup

12031=00300=5 base value units

11402=00400=3 base value units

### Relative value units for relative value order

12031=4.4 RVU

11402=3.29 RVU

### Overall anesthesiology code for the case for the billing anesthesiologist

00300-QY-P3, 36556

### Overall anesthesiology code for the case for the billing CRNA

00300-QX-P3

00300 Anesthesia for all procedures on the integumentary system, muscles, and nerves of the head, neck, and posterior trunk, not otherwise specified

### Units calculation

Total units=Base+Time+Physical status+Emergency=5.0+7.7+1+0=13.7

### Clinical viewpoint

The patient has a mass in the upper left chest overlying the head of the left clavicle, which upon pathological analysis turns out to be a benign neoplasm of peripheral nerves and autonomic nervous system of the thorax (ICD-10-CM code=D36.14). The patient requires excision of benign lesion including margins, excised diameter 1.1 to 2.0 cm (CPT code=11402) and repair, intermediate, wounds of the trunk (thorax), 2.5 cm or less (CPT code=12031). The overall anesthesiology code for the case is 00300, as determined by my anesthesiology coding method utilizing ASA Crosswalk Lookup. The CPT codes are in relative value order, based on highest relative value units (RVU) to lowest RVU. The anesthesiologist medically directed one CRNA for the case (see modifiers) and placed the non-tunneled central venous catheter (CPT code=36556) at the beginning of the case, not the CRNA.

## 27.

### Codes

70551, G93.40

### ASA Crosswalk Lookup

70551=7 base value units=01922

01922 Anesthesia for non-invasive imaging or radiation therapy

### Overall anesthesiology code for the case for the billing anesthesiologist

01922-QS-AA-P3, +99100

Units calculation=Base+Time+Physical status+Emergency (Qualifying circumstances)

For this Medicare patient, units calculation=Base=Time=7.0+3.0=10.0

Time units=45 (in minutes)/15=3.0

### Clinical viewpoint

This patient has encephalopathy, which is a severe systemic disease (PS III). The patient is a Medicare-insured patient (Medicare rules for age greater than 65) (+99100 Anesthesia for patient of extreme age) and therefore the units calculation for this Medicare-insured patient=Base+Time only. Note that on the actual CANPC exam, the total units calculated from the units calculation can round either up or down for the whole number for a value >= 0.5 incremental units.

## 28.

### Codes

74160, K46.9, D18.03

### Overall anesthesiology code for the billing anesthesiologist for the case

01922-QK-P3

### Overall anesthesiology code for the billing CRNAs for the case

01922-QX-P3

01922 Anesthesia for non-invasive imaging or radiation therapy

Units calculation=Base+Time+PS+Emergency (Qualifying circumstances) =7.0+3.7+1.0+0=11.7 (Can round up to 12.0 or down to 11.0 for the actual CANPC exam)

### Clinical viewpoint

The patient has an unspecified abdominal hernia and hemangioma of intra-abdominal structures as found on an abdominal CT scan with contrast (74160). The anesthesia is for non-invasive imaging (01922). In this case, note that the surgeon placed the central venous catheter at the beginning of the case. Because the surgeon placed the central venous catheter, the CPT code for central venous catheter placement is not included in the procedural coding for the case. The anesthesiologist medically directed 4 CRNAs in this case (modifier QK). For the actual CANPC exam, medically directing 4 CRNAs is the same as the medical direction of four concurrent anesthesia procedures involving qualified individuals (QK) as listed in the HCPCS II codebook.

## 29.

### Codes

64640-LT, G57.62

### ASA Crosswalk Lookup

64640=01991=3 base value units

01991 Anesthesia for diagnostic or therapeutic nerve blocks and injections; other than the prone position

### Overall anesthesia code for the billing CRNA

01991-QZ-P3, +99100, +99135

Units calculation (Medicare)=Base+Time =3.0+3.1=6.1

### Clinical viewpoint

In this case, the CRNA provides the anesthesia for the case without the help of an anesthesiologist (QZ). The patient undergoes destruction by neurolytic agent; other peripheral nerve or branch (64640) requiring general endotracheal anesthesia (01991). The patient is over 70 years old (+99100) and the anesthesia is complicated by the utilization of controlled hypotension. Note that the qualifying circumstances which I am calling "Emergency" affect the units calculation significantly.

## 30.

### Codes

29876-RT, 29881-RT, M23.221, M65.9, M94.261

### ASA Crosswalk

29876=01400=4 base value units

29881=01400=4 base value units

### Relative value order based on relative value units

29876=18.92 RVU

29881=15.56 RVU

### Overall anesthesiology code for the billing anesthesiologist

01400-QK-P3

### Overall anesthesiology code for the billing CRNA

01400-QX-P3

01400 Anesthesia for open or surgical arthroscopic procedures on knee joint; not otherwise specified

Units calculation=Base+Time+Physical status+Emergency=4.0+15.3+1.0+0=20.3

### Clinical viewpoint

The patient undergoes an arthroscopy, knee, surgical with synovectomy, major, 2 or more compartments (29876) and arthroscopy, knee, surgical with meniscectomy (medial AND lateral, including any meniscal shaving) including debridement/shaving of articular cartilage (chondroplasty), same or separate compartments, when performed (29880). The overall anesthesiology code for the case is 01400 Anesthesia for open or surgical arthroscopic procedures on the knee joint. There is a tie for the base value units in ASA Crosswalk Lookup, but the tie makes no difference. The corresponding anesthesia code for both 29876 and 29881 is 01400. In this case, the anesthesiologist is medically directing 2 CRNAs. This is how the information is written in the actual CANPC exam. Therefore, what to know about the actual CANPC exam is that QK Medical direction of two, three, or four concurrent anesthesia procedures involving qualified individuals means medically directing 2 CRNAs for this case.

## 31.

### Codes

57452, 99203-25, N87.9

### ASA Crosswalk Lookup

57452=00940=3 base value units

### Overall anesthesiology code for the case for the billing anesthesiologist

00940-AA-P3

00940 Anesthesia for vaginal procedures (including biopsy of labia, vagina, cervix, or endometrium); not otherwise specified

Units calculation=Base+Time+Physical status+Emergency=3.0+3.7+1.0+0=7.7 (Can round up to 8.0 or round down to 7.0 for actual CANPC exam; rounding up is the more correct answer in case both are listed)

### Clinical viewpoint

The patient underwent colposcopy (57452) for cervical dysplasia (N87.9). The encounter is an office visit for a new patient (99203). Modifier 25 is included for the procedure with an Evaluation and Management service. The general endotracheal anesthesia is for vaginal procedures (00940). The anesthesia services were performed personally by the anesthesiologist (AA) only. The patient has asthma with cervical dysplasia (N87.9).

## 32.

### Codes

57452, 56820, 99203-25, D07.1, K62.5

### ASA Crosswalk Lookup

57452=00940=3 base value units

56820=00940=3 base value units

### Relative value order based on relative value units

56820=2.49 RVU

57452=2.64 RVU

99203=2.17 RVU

### Overall anesthesiology code for the case for the billing CRNA

00940-QS-QZ-P3, +99140

+99140 Anesthesia complicated by emergency conditions

00940 Anesthesia for vaginal procedures (including biopsy of labia, vagina, cervix, or endometrium); not otherwise specified

Units calculation=Base+Time+Physical status+Emergency (Qualifying circumstances) =3.0+5.1+1.0+2.0=11.1 (Rounds to 11 or 12 for actual CANPC exam)

### Clinical viewpoint

The patient underwent colposcopy of the cervix including upper/adjacent vagina (57452) and colposcopy of the vulva (56820) for hemorrhage of anus and rectum (K62.5) which found carcinoma in situ of the vulva (D07.1). The anesthesia is a monitored anesthesia care service (modifier QS) complicated by the emergency condition of bleeding (+99140). What is the term "Emergency" is listed as qualifying circumstances in the units calculation. The anesthesia is for vaginal procedures (00940). The emergency condition (+99140) adds 2.0 units to the units calculation.

## 33.

### Codes

58100, 99213-25, R19.09

### ASA Crosswalk Lookup

58100=00940=3 base value units

### Relative value units for relative value order

58100=2.01 RVU

99213=1.44 RVU

### Overall anesthesiology code for the case for the billing anesthesiologist

00940-QY-P3, 36620-RT

### Overall anesthesiology code for the billing CRNA

00940-QX-P3

00940 Anesthesia for vaginal procedures (including biopsy of labia, vagina, cervix, or endometrium); not otherwise specified

Units calculation (for this Medicare-insured patient) =Base+Time=3.0+3.8=6.8 (Rounds to either 7.0 or 6.0 for actual CANPC exam; if both choices are possible, choose 7.0)

### Clinical viewpoint

The patient received a procedure of endometrial sampling (biopsy) (58100) with an established patient level 3 visit (99213-25) for an intra-abdominal and pelvic swelling, mass, and lump (R19.09). The endometrial biopsy was done for perimenopausal bleeding, but the results of the biopsy are still pending. Therefore, we are not able to identify the intra-abdominal and pelvic swelling, mass and lump in detail. The anesthesia is for vaginal procedures. The anesthesiologist placed a radial arterial catheter in the right artery at the beginning of the case. Therefore, 36620 is coded for the billing anesthesiologist. If the surgeon places a catheter at the beginning of the case, the procedure is not coded for the billing anesthesiologist.

## 34.

### Codes

52204, C67.4

### ASA Crosswalk

52204=00910=3 base value units

### Overall anesthesiology code for the case for the billing anesthesiologist

00910-AD-P4, +99135

### Overall anesthesiology code for the case for the billing CRNA

00910-QX, 36556-LT, +99135

00910 Anesthesia for transurethral procedures (including urethrocystoscopy); not otherwise specified

Units calculation=Base+Time+Physical status+Emergency (Qualifying circumstances) =3.0+9.7+2.0+5.0=19.7

### Clinical viewpoint

A cystourethroscopy with biopsies (52204) was performed which found malignant neoplasm of the posterior wall of the bladder (C67.4). Anesthesia was for transurethral procedures (00910). The anesthesiologist directed five CRNAs (modifier AD) for this case. A non-tunneled central venous catheter was placed in the left internal jugular vein (36556) by the CRNA. In this case, the anesthesia was complicated by utilization of controlled hypotension (+99135) as determined by the anesthesiologist. This finding added 5.0 units in what I call Emergency or qualifying circumstances to the total units calculation.

## 35.

### Codes

11424, 12041, T87.31, L72.0

### ASA Crosswalk Lookup

11424=00300=5 base value units

12041=00300=5 base value units

### Overall anesthesiology code for the billing anesthesiologist

00300-AA-P2, 93312, 93503

00300 Anesthesia for all procedures on the integumentary system, muscles, and nerves of the head, neck, and posterior trunk, not otherwise specified

Units calculation (Medicare)=Base+Time=5.0+15.9=20.9 (Can round up to 21 or down to 20 for actual CANPC exam; if both choices are listed, select 21)

### Clinical viewpoint

The patient underwent excision of a 2.2 cm diameter benign lesion including 0.5 cm margins, hands, 3.1 to 4.0 cm (11424) and intermediate repair of wounds of hands, 2.5 cm or less (2.25 cm) (12041). The anesthesia was for all procedures on the integumentary system, muscles, and nerves of the head, neck, and posterior trunk (00300). The anesthesiologist placed a Swanz-Ganz catheter (93503) at the beginning of the case and performed a transesophageal echocardiogram (93312) during the case. The codes count for the overall anesthesiology code for the case for the billing anesthesiologist since the anesthesiologist placed the catheter and performed the TEE. In this case, since it is not the procedure performed in the case (the reason for the surgery), 93503 and 93312 are not used in the ASA Crosswalk Lookup.

## 36.

### Codes

27829-RT, 27792-RT, S82.61XA, S93.431A, W19.XXXA, Y93.89, Y92.59, Y99.0

### ASA Crosswalk Lookup

27792=01480=3 base value units

27829=01480=3 base value units

### Overall anesthesiology code for the case for the billing anesthesiologist

01480-AA-P3, +99116

01480 Anesthesia for open procedures on bones of lower leg, ankle, and foot; not otherwise specified

Units calculation=Base+Time+Physical status+Emergency (qualifying circumstances) =3.0+10.5+1.0+5.0=19.5

Time units calculation=157/15=10.5

### Clinical viewpoint

Open treatment of a distal fibular fracture (lateral malleolus), includes internal fixation, when performed (27792) and open treatment of distal tibiofibular joint (syndesmosis) disruption, includes internal fixation, when performed (27829) were performed for these conditions. Anesthesia was for open procedures on bones of lower leg, ankle, and foot (01480). The injury occurred from a fall (W19.XXXA) at work (Y99.0). The anesthesia was complicated by the qualifying circumstance utilization of total body hypothermia (+99116). The qualifying circumstance added 5.0 units to the units calculation.

## 37.

### Codes

25111-LT, M67.432

### ASA Crosswalk Lookup

25111=01810=3 base value units

01810 Anesthesia for all procedures on nerves, muscles, tendons, fascia, and bursae of forearm, wrist, and hand

### Overall anesthesiology code for the case for the billing CRNA

01810-QS-QZ-P2

### Units calculation

Units calculation=Base+Time+Physical status+Emergency (Qualifying circumstances) =3.0+6.8+0+0=9.8 (Can round up to 10 or down to 9 for actual CANPC exam)

Time units=102/15=6.8

### Units calculation

The patient receives an excision of ganglion, wrist (dorsal or volar); recurrent (25111) for a ganglion of the wrist (M67.432). The anesthesia (01810) was for all procedures on nerves, muscles, tendons, fascia, and bursae of forearm, wrist, and hand. The anesthesia is monitored care service (modifier QS). Pathological analysis of the specimen obtained during surgery finds that the left wrist soft tissue mass that the patient presented with is a recurrent ganglion cyst.

## 38.

### Codes

28297-T5, M20.11, E11.9

### Overall anesthesia code for the case for the case for the billing anesthesiologist

99156, +99157 x 15

### Clinical viewpoint

The patient underwent Correction, hallux valgus (bunionectomy), with sesamoidectomy, when performed; with first metatarsal and medial cuneiform joint arthrodesis, any method (28297) for hallux valgus (acquired), right foot (M20.11). The patient also has diabetes (E11.9) and therefore has a physical status III. The patient underwent moderate conscious sedation with an intraservice time of 3:55 hours which is 235 minutes. The anesthesiologist performed the moderate conscious sedation (99156, +99157 x 15) for the case while the surgeon performed the surgery. The 235 minutes rounds up to 240 minutes for the final 15 minutes.

## 39.

### Codes

58660, N99.4

### ASA Crosswalk Lookup

58660=00840=6 base value units

### Overall anesthesiology code for the case for the billing anesthesiologist

00840-QY-P3, 36556-LT

### Overall anesthesiology code for the case for the billing CRNA

00840-QX-P3

00840 Anesthesia for intraperitoneal procedures in lower abdomen including laparoscopy; not otherwise specified

Units calculation=Base+Time+Physical status+Emergency=6.0+4.3+1.0+0=11.3

### Clinical viewpoint

The patient underwent laparoscopy, surgical; with the removal of adnexal structures (58660) for post-procedural pelvic peritoneal adhesions (N99.4). The anesthesiologist placed a central venous catheter in the patient before the surgery (36556-LT). The procedure was performed by the anesthesiologist and therefore counts in the anesthesia coding.

## 40.

### Codes

37765-LT, 37700-LT, I83.892

### ASA Crosswalk Lookup

37765=01520=3 base value units

37700=01265=3 base value units

### Overall anesthesiology code for the case for the billing anesthesiologist

01520-AD-P3, +99116

### Overall anesthesiology code for the billing CRNA

01520-QX-P3, +99116

01520 Anesthesia for procedures on veins of lower leg; not otherwise specified

Units calculation=Base+Time+Physical status+Emergency (Qualifying circumstances) =3.0+10.7+1.0+5.0=19.7

Time units calculation=160/15=10.7

### Clinical viewpoint

The patient received stab phlebectomy of varicose veins, 1 extremity; 10-20 stab incisions (37765) and ligation and division of long saphenous vein at the saphenofemoral junction, or distal interruptions (37700) for varicose veins of the left lower extremity with other complications (I83.892). In ASA Crosswalk Lookup, the base value units are tied. Based on relative value order as looked up in the Relative Value File 37765 is the first-listed CPT code. Therefore, 01520 is the overall anesthesia code for the case. The anesthesia was complicated by utilization of total body hypothermia, which adds 5.0 units in qualifying circumstances to the units calculation.

## 41.

### Codes

64721-RT, G56.01

### ASA Crosswalk Lookup

64721=01810=3 base value units

### Overall anesthesiology code for the case for the billing anesthesiologist

01810-G8-AA-P2, 36620

01810 Anesthesia for all procedures on nerves, muscles, tendons, fascia, and bursae of forearm, wrist, and hand

Units calculation (Medicare patient) =Base+Time+Physical status+Emergency (qualifying circumstances) =3.0+4.5=7.5

### Clinical viewpoint

The patient underwent a neuroplasty and/or transposition; median nerve at carpal tunnel (64721) for carpal tunnel syndrome, right upper limb (G56.01). The anesthesia (01810) was monitored anesthesia care for a deep complex, complicated, or markedly invasive surgical procedure (modifier G8).

## 42.

### Codes

27603-RT, S80.11XD

### ASA Crosswalk Lookup

27603=01470=3 base value units

### Overall anesthesiology code for the billing anesthesiologist

01470-AA-P2, +99140

01470 Anesthesia for procedures on nerves, muscles, tendons, and fascia of the lower leg, ankle, and foot; not otherwise specified

Units calculation=Base+Time+Physical status+Emergency (Qualifying circumstances) =3.0+1.8+0+2.0=6.8

### Clinical viewpoint

The patient underwent Incision and drainage, leg or ankle; deep abscess or hematoma (27603) for contusion of the right lower leg (S80.11). The patient had emergency bleeding during the surgery. Therefore, the anesthesia was complicated by emergency conditions (+99140).

## 43.

### Codes

54161, N47.6, N47.1

### ASA Crosswalk Lookup

54161=00920=3 base value units

### Overall anesthesiology code for the case for the billing anesthesiologist

00920-QY-P2

### Overall anesthesiology code for the case for the billing CRNA

00920-QX-P2

00920 Anesthesia for procedures on male genitalia (including open urethral procedures); not otherwise specified

Units calculation=Base+Time+Physical status+Emergency (Qualifying circumstances) =3.0+3.1+0+0=6.1

Time units calculation=47/15=3.1

### Clinical viewpoint

The patient underwent circumcision, surgical excision other than clamp, device, or dorsal slit; older than 28 days of age (54161) for balanoposthitis (N47.6) and phimosis (N47.1). The patient is 12 years old and therefore the CPT code 54161 is the correct choice for this circumcision.

## 44.

### Codes

10140, T81.42XA, Z86.14

### ASA Crosswalk Lookup

10140=00400=3 base value units

## Overall anesthesiology code for the case for the billing anesthesiologist

00400-AA-P3, +99140

00400 Anesthesia for procedures on the integumentary system on the extremities, anterior trunk, and perineum; not otherwise specified

Units calculation=Base+Time+Physical status+Emergency (Qualifying circumstances) =3.0+11.0+1.0+2.0=17.0

Time units calculation=165/15=11.0

## Clinical viewpoint

The patient underwent incision and drainage of hematoma; seroma or fluid collection (10140) for infection following a procedure, deep incisional surgical site (T81.42XA). The patient has a personal history of Methicillin-resistant Staphylococcus aureus infection (Z86.14). The patient is status post lumbar laminectomy L5 bilateral, recent surgery and has deep seroma formation and drainage of serous fluid from the incisional site. The anesthesia was complicated by the emergency condition of bleeding (+99140), which adds 2.0 units to the units calculation. A P.I.C.C. line was in place at the beginning of the case as placed by a surgeon prior to the surgery and therefore does not count as a CPT code.

# 45.

## Codes

66183-RT, E11.9, I10, H40.2212

## ASA Crosswalk Lookup

66183=00140=5 base value units

## Overall anesthesiology code for the case for the billing anesthesiologist

00140-AA-P3

00140 Anesthesia for procedures on the eye; not otherwise specified

Units calculation=Base+Time+Physical status+Emergency (Qualifying circumstances) =5.0+9.3+1.0+0=15.3

## Clinical viewpoint

The anesthesia is for procedures on the eye; not otherwise specified (00140). The patient has chronic angle-closure glaucoma, moderate stage right eye. The patient also has diabetes type II and hypertension (physical status III).

# 46.

## Codes

38500-LT, C85.95, E11.9

## ASA Crosswalk Lookup

38500=01610=5 base value units

### Overall anesthesiology code for the case for the billing anesthesiologist

01610-QY-P3

### Overall anesthesiology code for the case for the billing anesthesiologist

01610-QX-P3, 36620-RT

01610 Anesthesia for all procedures on nerves, muscles, tendons, fascia, and bursae of shoulder and axilla

Units calculation=Base+Time+Physical status+Emergency (Qualifying circumstances) =5.0+5.7+1.0+0=11.7

Time units calculation=85/15=5.7

### Clinical viewpoint

The patient underwent biopsy or excision of lymph node(s); open, superficial (38500) for a condition confirmed to be Non-Hodgkin lymphoma, unspecified, lymph nodes of inguinal region and lower limb (C85.95). Anesthesia was performed for all procedures on nerves, muscles, tendons, fascia, and bursae of shoulder and axilla (01610). A central venous catheter was placed at the beginning of the case by the CRNA (36620-RT). A central venous catheter, radial arterial catheter, Swan Ganz catheter or TEE (trans-esophageal echocardiogram) placed or performed at the beginning of the case by the anesthesiologist, CRNA, but not the surgeon counts as a CPT code reported in the overall anesthesiology code for the case.

## 47.

### Codes

49560, K43.2

### ASA Crosswalk Lookup

49560=00752=6 base value units

### Overall anesthesiology code for the case for the billing anesthesiologist

00752-AA-P2, 36556-LT

00752 Anesthesia for hernia repairs in upper abdomen; lumbar and ventral (incisional) hernias and/or wound dehiscence

Units calculation=Base+Time+Physical status+Emergency (Qualifying circumstances)=6.0+9.1+0+0=15.1

### Clinical viewpoint

The patient underwent repair of initial incisional or ventral hernia; reducible (49560) for incisional hernia without obstruction or gangrene (K43.2). The anesthesiologist placed a central venous catheter in the left internal jugular vein (36556-LT) at the beginning of the case. Therefore, the code counts for the overall anesthesiology code for the billing anesthesiologist.

## 48.

### Codes

12032, 99283-25, S61.216A

### ASA Crosswalk Lookup

12032=00300=5 base value units

### Overall anesthesiology code for the case for the billing anesthesiologist

00300-QZ-P3, +99140

00300 Anesthesia for all procedures on the integumentary system, muscles, and nerves of the head, neck, and posterior trunk, not otherwise specified

### Clinical viewpoint

The CRNA personally provided the general endotracheal anesthesia for the case (modifier QZ). The anesthesia was complicated by emergency conditions of emergency bleeding (+99140).

## 49.

### Codes

0232-LT, 20680-LT, T84.84XA

### ASA Crosswalk Lookup

20680=01360=5 base value units

### Overall anesthesiology code for the case for the billing anesthesiologist

01360-AA-P3

01360 Anesthesia for open procedures on lower one-third of the femur

Units calculation (for Medicare patient)=Base+Time=5.0+19.1=24.1

Time=287/15=19.1

### Clinical viewpoint

Removal of the implant; deep (eq. buried wire, pin, screw, metal band, nail, rod, or plate) (20680) for pain due to internal orthopedic prosthetic devices, implants, and grafts (T84.84XA). The patient is a Medicare patient, and therefore the units calculation is =Base+Time only.

## 50.

### Codes

27814-LT, S82.842A

### ASA Crosswalk Lookup

27814=01480=3 base value units

Left femoral block

64447-LT

### Overall anesthesiology code for the case for the billing anesthesiologist

01480-QK-P3, 64447-LT, 36556-LT

### Overall anesthesiology code for the case for the billing CRNA

01480-QX-P3, 64447-LT

01480 Anesthesia for open procedures on bones of lower leg, ankle, and foot; not otherwise specified

Units calculation=Base+Time+Physical status+Emergency (Qualifying circumstances)=3.0+11.8+1.0+0=15.8

Time=177/15=11.8

### Clinical viewpoint

The anesthesia was general endotracheal anesthesia combined with a femoral block. Therefore, both codes for the general endotracheal anesthesia and femoral block are coded. Anesthesia (01480) was for open procedures on bones of lower leg, ankle, and foot; not otherwise specified. A left femoral block is an Injection, anesthetic agent; femoral nerve, single (64447). A central venous catheter was placed into the left internal jugular vein (36556-LT) by the anesthesiologist at the beginning of the case, and therefore the CPT code counts in the overall anesthesiology code for the billing anesthesiologist.

# References

The author gratefully acknowledges that the cases used in this book were sourced from the following excellent references and were modified to add more details and clarity. These references are reputable in the healthcare field; the users of this book will find them extremely helpful in preparing for various medical coding certification exams. The readers are recommended to study these resources for preparation of certification examinations and career enhancement as medical administrators, coders, and billers. Cases 1-25, for the texts, were sourced from Professional Coding Practice from AHIMA and modified by the author. Cases 26-50, for the texts, were sourced from 2018 Practicode COC-A ICD-10 Practicum from American Academy of Professional Coders, and modified by the author. The coding solutions (provided towards the end), anesthesia and pain management coding, units calculation, and clinical viewpoints are written by the author and based on his original work.


American Health Information Management Association. *Clinical Coding Workout: Practice Exercises for Skill Development, without Online Answers, 2016*. AHIMA Press, 20160201. VitalBook file.

American Health Information Management Association. *Virtual CCS-P Prep.*, 2018.

American Health Information Management Association. *Professional Coding Practice*. AHIMA Press, 2018.

Optum360. *2017 ICD-10-CM Coding Workbook for Cardiology*. Optum360, LLC, 2016.

Optum360, *2016 ICD-10-CM Coding Workbook for General Surgery*. Optum360, LLC, 2015.

COC-A ICD-10 Practicum, 2018. Practicode. American Academy of Professional Coders, Salt Lake City, UT, 2018.

An Insider's View: Field Avoidance and Special Positioning, American Academy of Professional Coders, Salt Lake City, UT, 2017

Merriam Webster's Medical Desk Dictionary, Merriam-Webster Incorporated, Clifton Park, NY, 2005

2016-2017 AHA Coding Clinic in ICD-10-CM/PCS and HCPCS, American Hospital Association (AHA), Chicago, IL, 2017.

2018 Official CPC Certification Study Guide, American Academy of Professional Coders, Salt Lake City, UT, 2018.

CPT Professional 2019

HCPCS Level II Expert 2019

ICD-10-CM 2019

2019 ASA (American Society of Anesthesiologists) Crosswalk®

2019 ASA Relative Value Guide®

2019 National Physician Fee Schedule Relative Value File January Release copyrighted by 2017 American Medical Association and 2018/19 American Dental Association

PFS Relative Value Files 2019 RVU19A

www.cms.gov

# Author's Background

Vino C. Mody Jr. has worked in the healthcare field for 15 years at different hospitals in the U.S. and Sweden. He completed medical coding specialist certificate programs from the University of Georgia and U.S. Career Institute, and a CPMA course from the American Academy of Professional Coders. Vino has achieved several important coding and billing certifications (COC, CPC, CCS-P, CANPC, CCVTC, CEDC, CMAA, CBCS, 4Med CICP, and RMC)*. He has worked as a coding instructor and a coder for three years in health care institutes and with coding consultants in El Paso, Texas. He is presently working in the medical administration department at Mesa Hills Hospital in El Paso, Texas, where he performs coding, medical auditing, medical transcription, quality data analysis, and surgery coding. He also runs a medicine service, resolves billing issues, and coordinates resolution of health information software issues. He has also completed a pharmacology and pharmaceutical sales training course, earning Certified National Pharmaceutical Representative (CNPR) certification. He has a Certified Risk Management Consultant (CRMC) certification from a confidential Texas corporation.

Vino has ten years of experience in the field of medicine, along with a medical degree from Emory University School of Medicine in Atlanta, Georgia. He has received medical training from Yale-New Haven Hospital (Waterbury, Connecticut) and Brown University/Lifespan (Providence, Rhode Island).

Vino has a Licentiate degree and Ph.D. from Karolinska Institutet in Stockholm, Sweden, combined with eight years of experience in ophthalmology research and teaching. His subjects of research included ophthalmology, surgery, medicine, and pediatrics. Vino was a clinical researcher for Karolinska Institutet for eight years and has published 25 original publications and 100 conference abstracts. Vino also served as the proctor for the National Board of Examiners in Optometry (NBEO) for three years and as editor of three different basic science clinical research journals at Karolinska in Sweden. He obtained his Bachelor's degree in molecular biology from Vanderbilt University in Nashville, Tennessee, graduating Summa Cum Laude.

Vino enjoys tennis and has played for the Parkview High School Tennis Team in Georgia and the Atlanta Lawn Tennis Association (ALTA) during his academic years in Georgia.

Please refer to website www.medpracticeprocess.com for more details on Vino Mody, Jr.'s background and services provided by him.

# *Acronyms

| | | |
|---|---|---|
| COC | - | Certified Outpatient Coder |
| CPC | - | Certified Professional Coder |
| CCS-P | - | Certified Coding Specialist-Physician based |
| CANPC | - | Certified Anesthesia and Pain management Coder |
| CCVTC | - | Certified Cardiovascular and Thoracic surgery Coder |
| CEDC | - | Certified Emergency Department Coder |
| CMAA | - | Certified Medical Administrative Assistant |
| CBCS | - | Certified Billing and Coding Specialist |
| 4Med CICP | - | Certificate of ICD-10-CM Proficiency |
| RMC | - | Registered medical coder |